AT THE
CLOSE
OF
DAY

A Person-Centered Guidebook
on End-of-Life Care

Lance L. Davis, MD MPH &
Albert H. Keller, DMin

At the Close of Day: A Person-Centered Guidebook for End-of-Life Care

ISBN 0-9753488-0-9
Library of Congress Control Number: 2004093829

Copyright © 2004
Lance L. Davis, MD, MPH and Albert H. Keller, DMin

Printed by Gorham Printing, Rochester, Washington USA
Cover and book design: Kathryn Campbell
Editor: Barbara J. Fandrich
Assistant Editor: Corrinne Norman, MAT

This book is published in a grassroots fashion. The authors maintained
complete control of the content in order to protect the integrity and honesty of the information herein. It is not intended to replace normal medical care or relationships with health care professionals; rather, it should
complement those relationships and foster communication.

www.atthecloseofday.com

AT *the* CLOSE *of* DAY

This book is dedicated to the patients
and their families who have allowed us to share
in their dying process. Their stories and experiences
have allowed us to pass this information on to others.

FOREWORD

I feel very privileged to place my endorsement on this work. Over the years, I have had many discussions about the dying process with Dr. Davis and Dr. Keller. I know they both have approached this work in a thoughtful, comprehensive manner. More importantly, they have approached this work with zeal because of the need they feel to disseminate this information to the people who need it most. The final product is a great resource for many individuals and families facing some of life's most difficult problems. I know the authors are proud of the end result, and I am proud to endorse it.

Dr. Davis and I went to medical school together and over the years have had many opportunities to discuss what our health care system does well and the things it does poorly. It's clear that the health system in the United States is without peer when it comes to technological and pharmacological innovation. No other country in the world expends such energy and expense in heroic medicine on the sickest in society. However, this success comes at a price, and the price we pay as a society is twofold. First, and perhaps the easiest to correct with public policy, is the shifting of vast resources to health care that has its impact on relatively few individuals. We do not invest resources on combating tobacco abuse and obesity, on opening up universal basic primary care, and on preventative medicine, but rather we spend that money in often-futile exercises of intensive care. However, the more insidious price we pay as a society is one of attitude. The successes of medicine in the twenty-first century have led a majority of people to believe that doctors, nurses, and hospitals can cure every ill. This belief system plays a cruel joke on all of us by forcing patients to request, and their doctors to give, care that is not only futile, but also often detrimental to the patient's best interest. This book that Dr. Davis and Dr. Keller have written goes a long way toward addressing this belief system that has become ingrained in all of us to a greater or lesser extent.

As the authors caution at the beginning of the book, many maladies that were once incurable, such as Hodgkin's lymphoma and testicular cancer, are now curable. Decisions regarding care should always be made in conjunction with a physician who is knowledgeable in the field. However, once it is known that further interventions will only lead to more suffering, this book is an invaluable aid. As a practicing hematologist, oncologist, and palliative care physician, I work with patients every day who are facing formidable illnesses. I wish I could devote the hours that it takes to fully discuss and explore all of the complex problems of patients going through the dying process with them and their families. The fact of the matter is that although I would like to spend these hours with each patient, I simply don't have the time. I am glad I have this book as a resource that my patients can read at their leisure. With its conversational format and straightforward language, it addresses in depth many of the issues that face the sickest among us. Often, families don't feel comfortable asking many of these difficult questions in front of their loved ones, or they forget their questions when they visit their doctors. This book, which can be easily read in one sitting, touches on the questions that frequently come up when someone is facing the prospect of death. It does not use a "one size fits all" approach to *The Active Management of Dying*, but rather recognizes that cultural and experiential differences can be crucial when one is wrestling with these difficult problems.

I particularly like the use of real life examples. As I read this book I recognized in these examples many of the same situations that face my own patients. Although every patient is unique, I know that many people reading this book will see their own situations mirrored in the examples presented. The authors very skillfully present complex psychological discussions in easy-to-understand language. They work through these discussions in much the same way that I talk to my patients, with each concept building up to the next. However, the most important part of this book is the practical information that it presents. The authors give their readers information on how to get things done and advice on how to navigate the foreign waters of health care.

I highly recommend this book to any person or family facing death and dying. These times are the most challenging in any life, and this book is an invaluable resource that I hope will reach many, many people.

Jerry W. Mitchell Jr., MD
Associate Director of Palliative Care
Grant Hospital, Columbus, Ohio
Board certified: Internal Medicine, Hematology, and Oncology

THE STORY

OF A DOCTOR

AND A PATIENT

Lance writes...

There she lay, eighty-seven years old and weighing less than ninety pounds. It was 3:00 AM, and I was the attending physician at the county hospital's emergency department (ED) in Charleston, South Carolina. Due to a series of crippling strokes, Dorothy P. had been bed-bound for years, and her family had provided all her basic needs. Before her family brought her to the ED that night, she had refused food completely for three weeks. During the several months prior to that, she had taken only a little nourishment, despite her family's best attempts to feed her. That night she had begun to slip away. Her family panicked and called an ambulance.

After taking a history, conducting an exam, and checking her lab work, I realized she was dying. After years of training and experience, I knew the scenario and the task ahead all too well. I met with the family and helped them understand the process. Hospice was contacted, and she was allowed to go home, where she would spend her final hours.

Despite years of experience and hundreds of similar cases, I still get inwardly anxious when I approach a patient or family to recommend the transition from therapeutic intervention to comfort care. It is a tremendous and unsettling responsibility, as well as an opportunity to improve an otherwise difficult situation. I will never be able to predict the precise moment when a person will die. At the same time, once I recognize medical futility, I am committed to assisting terminal patients to achieve a peaceful, dignified death.

Three days later Dorothy P.'s obituary appeared. I telephoned her home and spoke to her daughter. (I actually had called during the wake.) Her daughter said she had passed away quietly and comfortably in her own bed, and the family was coping well. I knew in that moment the right decision had been made. I also knew it was time to get serious about writing this book.

HOW TO USE
THIS BOOK

Although we set out to write a guidebook, each reader will derive something different from reading this book, and we hope it will nourish genuine growth and change. The book is designed to be your professional consultation with a doctor, Lance L. Davis, MD, MPH, and an ethicist, Albert H. Keller, DMin. You will notice that many sections are introduced by a phrase saying either "Lance writes . . ." or "Bert writes. . . ." Keep in mind that Lance writes from the perspective of a physician, and Bert writes from the perspective of an ethicist and pastor. We invite you to envision yourself at a table having a three-way conversation with the authors.

Our overall goal is to help you develop a plan to manage the dying process, whether you are a patient, family member, or health care professional. Although the book is primarily for the layperson, we believe health care professionals and students will also find it to be a valuable tool. Information about the authors is available at the end of the book.

If you read the book from start to finish, you will find yourself moving through several stages of awareness and understanding. If you use the text as a reference for specific issues, you will also gather important information but may not understand the whole perspective that we offer.

This print version and the audio version are both suitable as independent resources. However, we believe the concurrent use of the audio version (which would serve as a focus for family meetings) and the print version (for individual reference and reflection) would be of greatest benefit as you develop your knowledge and plans.

As you read through these pages, please note that the situations apply equally to men and women—we have alternated male and female gender in order to balance the examples.

TABLE OF CONTENTS

ACKNOWLEDGMENTS

This book is written primarily from the hearts and minds of Bert Keller and Lance Davis, with very few references. However, in order to gain the experience and comfort to speak frankly and confidently about death "from the hip," a multitude of teachers, mentors, colleagues, friends, and patients contributed to each author's views, opinions, and expertise.

We would specifically like to thank the Department of Family Medicine at the Medical University of South Carolina in Charleston for providing a forum for education and sharing of ideas.

A special thanks is given to Jonathan Sack, MD, who never stops asking perhaps the most pertinent question in medicine today, "Are we treating the patient or ourselves?"

Recognition and thanks go to David Garr, MD, for sharing a story about the death of his own father, in order to sensitize the resident physicians under his tutelage.

Medical education itself is a public domain. Even doctors who went to private medical schools receive, at some point, education and training that the public has funded in some form. Therefore, medical knowledge is not a possession that can be claimed or owned by any individual. Instead, it is a public trust to be used and shared responsibly. We share in it, we refine it, we hopefully use it to the betterment of our patients and communities, and then we pass it on. Therefore, each one of us has a proud stake in the contributions of medical educators and health care professionals. Lay readers themselves deserve a measure of thanks for contributions to this work.

We appreciate the patient stewardship provided by our editors, Barbara Fandrich and Corrinne Norman, MAT, who saw the vision and kept it going even when the authors were growing weary.

Many thanks go to Jerry Mitchell, MD, who understood exactly what we wanted to do with this work and added valuable insights at every turn.

Finally, to those who purchased the initial manuscript of this text while it was still rough, for their constructive feedback and comments, which helped guide us to the first print edition, we give hearty thanks and sincere wishes that the information proved useful and comforting.

The Active
Management *of* Dying

Lance writes . . .

The reader should understand this book is written to address the needs of people who have reached the point where prolonging the basic life functions will not result in meaningful quality of life. These are people who have undergone proper medical evaluation and treatment in an attempt to restore them to health, but for whom treatment of the disease is not working any longer. Bear in mind that the newly diagnosed patient may have many options. Many people with life-threatening diseases can benefit from proper therapy and can return to a state of good health. If the time comes, though, when curative treatment is no longer achieving its goal, then the person enters another phase of treatment called *palliative,* or comfort care.

When Bert Keller and I sat down to plan this book, I told him this was something I had to do. To me, it was like seeing a child in need of rescue, and having the means to achieve that rescue. One's duty would be clear and irresistible at that point. If one knows there is a serious problem and a definite way to help, then there is a compulsion to do something about it. That is my feeling about the care of the dying. I must admit it is not the happiest subject in the world. I never envisioned it as the topic of my first book. It is not even a topic I want to spend most of my time thinking about or dealing with. In that regard, I am like most other people. We want to live happy and productive lives, and we do not want to think about death. However, when we live in denial of death, without thinking or planning, death easily becomes a chaotic time, and the dying process becomes much more anxiety-provoking and more painful than it has to be.

Death, if it is well planned, can be a peaceful process. Once one accepts that idea, the fear of death and dying are diminished. People have a natural tendency to fear the unknown, but good planning can lessen that fear and make the experience better overall. For example, think of childbirth classes. Mothers who are well prepared, and who have birth plans, tend to have more comfortable and calm deliveries, as compared to mothers who have no prenatal education or training. The same can be said for most human endeavors, from camping trips to theatrical productions. The dying process is no different. Entering the experience with knowledge and planning makes the entire procedure smoother. We want to help you, the reader, come to terms with certain realities involved with death and dying, to be able to understand how people can die peacefully and comfortably in this society. We want to give you concrete tools to help yourself and those you care about to achieve "a good death," when that inevitable time occurs.

I tend to be a fun-loving guy. A friend once told me that I "eat life in large gulps." I like that view of myself. I am not a gloom-and-doom person. I began my career in medicine simply as a person who felt very fortunate to have a chance to help others.

During my years in college and medical school, we frequently discussed the topic of dying, especially in the context of American society.

I became aware of many problems and shortcomings that exist within our highly advanced medical system, but it was not until my residency in Family Medicine, coupled with long hours of work in various emergency departments, that I really began to see people dying on a regular basis. Through those experiences I began to understand some of the problems people experience during the dying process. Through professional experiences, as well as personal experiences within my own family, it became clear that most of us share the same range of emotions regarding mortality. I went through my own denial, resistance, fear, sadness, and other emotions that a human being feels when exposed to the death of human beings.

I have had many wise mentors along the way, and the coauthor of this book, Dr. Bert Keller, is in the forefront of those. To all of them I am deeply indebted. It was their guidance that helped to turn fear into motivation and powerlessness into action. They taught me to see through the myths and denial, allowing me to look at the reality of the process, so I could be of maximum assistance to the dying person in the hour of need. They taught me the actual knowledge and skills required to prevent undue suffering. Many of these lessons were tough to take, as I had always fantasized about saving lives, not accepting the finality of death. Yet, without such guidance, I would have been lost in those moments when medical futility was certain, death was near, and a human being lay before me in pain. It occurred to me that most other people have much less guidance and mentorship when it comes to dying in our society. Writing this book and offering guidance and mentorship to the reader was beyond a privilege, it was a duty and an honor. It is in this spirit that I share my reflections with the reader. I suspect that Bert shares some of the same motivation.

This book addresses situations where people actually go through a dying process. In other words, they suffer from disease, injury, or advanced age, which debilitates them and steals away their vital processes.

Some people die under traumatic or rapid circumstances and do not undergo a definable dying process. This book will relate less directly to those situations, but may be very helpful to the families left behind. *Please note: it is not intended for those who have been newly diagnosed with a serious illness, as many useful treatments exist for a wide variety of conditions that were once fatal.*

As I assemble my thoughts for this book, I envision late-stage cancer patients who have not responded to therapies; demented or neurologically devastated people who are bed-bound and unable to care for themselves; or those who have advanced heart or lung diseases for which there are no more useful treatments. These are all examples, and there are many others, of people for whom medical intervention has become futile. In other words, there are no further cures, and any further interventions such as breathing tubes, feeding tubes, artificial fluid administration, and medical or surgical therapies will do nothing except prolong life without adding any quality. For these people, further medical interventions may even prolong pain and suffering, and in the worse case, actually increase them. As a physician, I am bound to "First, do no harm." This is a serious charge. There are times when trying to help someone can actually cause harm. One must learn to recognize these situations and deal with them wisely.

None of this is meant to ignore the wondrous lifesaving interventions that modern medicine has to offer. There are, of course, many people who have been at death's door, then have been brought back from the brink to lead full lives afterward. Every physician dreams of having a chance to make a difference in these cases. However, as of today, death is inevitable, and each person will eventually reach a point where medical care is futile. When that point is reached and recognized, the greatest gift that can be given to the person is to be kept comfortable, to be nurtured and cared for, and not to experience unnecessary pain. It is during these times that spiritual needs and the concerns of the families can be addressed. When medical futility is recognized and accepted, the focus can shift away from unproductive medical interventions to highly productive comfort measures and palliative care.

Serious problems arise when futility has been reached but it is not recognized. I have watched many times as patients who would not benefit from life-prolonging measures were subjected to these interventions, and families were filled with false hopes and expectations. The patients suffered unnecessarily, and then still met their inevitable death. Optimally, each person should receive the type of care that best suits his or her individual situation. Those with potential for survival and recovery should receive appropriate intervention and treatment. Those who have no potential for recovery and meaningful survival should receive comfort care as their lives fade.

We invite you to read this book carefully, to reflect on the contents and case examples, to discuss it with your friends and family. It may awaken certain feelings in you, such as fear, anger, and denial. It is healthy and normal to experience a wide array of feelings when considering death. You will move through those feelings; do not run from them. Confront and work through them. Learn to think productively about what you and/or your loved ones might want during the dying process. Odds are that you bought this book because the dying process is currently affecting you or someone in your immediate circle. If so, you may be experiencing a wide range of emotions, and perhaps you are struggling to come up with the "right" way to respond. Although there is probably no right or wrong way, we hope this text will help you to develop strategies and skills to help you negotiate the dying process with a sense of relative confidence and peace.

As I write this brief introduction, last night's conversation with a close friend is fresh in my mind. My friend's father died in the early hours of the morning yesterday. His father was diagnosed with leukemia eight years ago, in his mid-seventies, but he did well and continued to go in to his law office every day until two weeks before his death. That's when the doctor told him his leukemia was active again and the end was near. The family enrolled him in hospice, and he remained at home, where his doctor called on him.

My friend told me the story of his father's final days and his death, which was peaceful and anticipated. He spoke of how achingly he would miss his father. He said something like this: "No man could have been a better father. He kept every promise he ever made to me. We both made mistakes and had difficult times, but we loved each other extravagantly, and in all the essentials my father was always there for me. A few days ago I sat down and wrote my father a four-page letter, telling him how much he meant to me. I read it to him—his consciousness was already slipping, but I think he understood. I have written him letters over the years, probably one a year, to tell him the same thing, even though I see him almost every day. Mother told me that they meant a great deal to him. I will miss him every day for the rest of my life, but there are no regrets. Nothing was left unsaid between us."

Questions for Reflection

At this point, it would be productive for you to pause and ask yourself the following questions, and then discuss them with family and close friends:

1. Do I believe people live forever?

2. If someone is obviously near the end of life, and prolongation of life will add no meaningful quality to that life, what is the best way to help that person?

3. When we offer futile medical interventions to someone who is in the dying process, who are we really treating, the patient or ourselves? Are we trying to make the patient feel better, or to make ourselves feel better?

4. How guilty would I feel if I had to give permission for someone else to die, if it was clear the person was at the end of his or her natural life?

5. How much do I think about death? Do I fear death? Do I fear seeing death?

6. Do I believe doctors work miracles or do they simply have skills and tools to help within the scope of the patient's natural health and abilities?

7. Which is closer to "playing God"—allowing someone to die peacefully and comfortably of natural causes, or temporarily preventing an imminent death using artificial means?

8. Have I discussed any of these issues with the people close to me?

These are difficult questions, and it would be a good idea for you to review them and really think about your feelings. There are no right or wrong answers, but these subjects set the stage for our discussion.

Death: Well-Managed vs. Chaotic

Lance writes . . .

The best place to start is by defining the goal. Since death is inevitable, it would be reasonable to develop a vision of an ideal, peaceful death. Then, we could work toward making it a reality.

Most people, if given a choice, would prefer to die of natural causes, in a comfortable place they call home, surrounded by people and things they know and love, and without pain, fear, or distress. Many of us want to die in our sleep, or at least in a peaceful state of mind. We want to know our spiritual concerns are taken care of, our family's grief would heal after our passing, and that by our being here the world had become a better place. We want our lives to feel well-lived and complete, and to have a sense of purpose and closure. In many cases, we can increase the likelihood of achieving an ideal death through fearless communication and good planning.

Now, let us look at the opposite situation. Very few of us want to die alone, in pain, tormented, or in a strange place. Normally, we do not want to have to undergo painful medical procedures if we are going to die relatively soon anyway. We do not want our families to feel guilty about decisions they have to make for us, and we do not want to feel we are overly burdening those who are caring for us.

Unfortunately, many people end up dying with these undesirable events unfolding. It saddens me greatly to know how frequently this type of death occurs. In many cases it could have gone much better. It is a nightmarish reality to know there are people who lie in nursing homes, kept alive by artificial feeding, who cannot control their bodily processes and cannot express their wants and desires. They cannot get out of bed. They develop painful sores. They waste away. They may even exhaust finances that represent an entire lifetime's worth of work and savings that they wanted to leave to their children or grandchildren. Sometimes they are not allowed to die even when it is clear they are emotionally and physically ready.

The stark contrast between these two realities is obvious. Most of us would choose the first scenario above rather than the second unfortunate reality. Ironically, very few people actively plan for the ideal death and, without planning, the chaotic death often occurs. This can be avoided by proper foresight on the part of the dying person, along with his or her family, medical providers, and support agencies.

As we move through this book, let us keep the well-managed death in mind as the goal toward which we work. Again, some people will die suddenly in traumatic and accidental cases. Others will die suddenly of rapid heart attacks or aneurysms in the brain. There are, of course, many unforeseen circumstances of death, but I contend that foresight and planning could even improve some of these situations.

Principles of The Active Management of Dying

I will now share with you a series of principles that I call *The Active Management of Dying.* I developed this concept during my residency to help me stay focused as I moved through the confusing territory of end-of-life planning. I find that these principles are broad enough to be used in almost every situation in which my patients and their families are facing the dying process, whether death was very near or more remote. These principles are applicable to everyone, not just to health care professionals. They tend to be most valuable when all members of the team are aware of them and are working together to ensure that each has been addressed. The principles of *The Active Management of Dying* serve as a 'big picture checklist' to help us stay on our path, and we will refer back to them throughout the book.

1. Accept the reality of the situation.

2. Identify the decision-makers.

3. Discuss the ultimate goals of care.

4. Create an end-of-life care plan.

5. Implement the care plan you created.

Bear in mind that these principles are applicable to dying persons, their families and caregivers, and to health care professionals. They can be applied in any setting, such as at home, in the hospital, in the emergency department, and in the nursing home or hospice house.

Notes

1

Accept *the* Reality *of the* Situation

Moving Through Fear to Hope

Bert writes ...

Imagine with me a person who has known, for a short time or a long time, that she has a life-threatening illness. Today the medical staff has told her that the chemotherapy, radiation therapy, or other treatment to stop the disease isn't working. She receives that information without evasion. Now she begins to reset her mind from the goal of recovery to the goal of dying well. Just as she found the strength necessary to fight the disease, she knows she will find the strength necessary to accept her condition with hope and peace.

Many readers will say, "Wait, that's not me. I'm not there yet—I'm far from being easy in my mind. Where does anyone find that kind of strength at such an extreme time as this? How can someone come to face death with that accepting attitude?" That's very honest. In this chapter, we will begin in an entirely different place, a place where fear dominates. We will then move step-by-step *from fear to hope*, to a place where death can be accepted and peace found. Please take this pilgrimage with me.

The memory of a chilling scene comes back to me as I start this journey. One winter night in 1972, a time when the Cold War seemed to be at its worst, I was on the night train from Warsaw to Berlin and was approaching the East German border. I hadn't been able to secure a visa to enter East Germany, but my Polish visa expired that day. I realized I had to get moving and take my chances. The train reached the international border at the Oder River about four o'clock in the morning. The Polish engines disengaged from the international passenger cars with a series of jolts, and we were suspended, lifeless, with no power source. After a long wait, East German soldiers, aggressively armed, boarded the train in the darkness and began checking travelers' official papers with flashlights. I felt a paralyzing dread take over my body. Even if I could speak the language (I could manage only a few basic words), what would I say? I wished I were anywhere else on earth than this dark river-border between one country that was pushing me out and another country where I was completely alone, without proper papers, and powerless.

When we are dying or when we accompany another who is close to the end of life, we approach an awesome boundary that we cannot see beyond. In modern American culture where most of us live, old pathways and treaties that used to point the way across that final border are largely unused these days. Many of us find ourselves making a pathway through terrain that is unknown, lonely, and frightening, and where we realize we are no longer in control. Maybe that's the most frightening thing of all: we have lost the sense of control over our life. Control is out of our hands. However skillful we've been before in taking care of ourselves and our affairs, maybe even exercising our will in broader spheres such as politics or commerce, that's irrelevant now. We are here not because we want to be but because we have to be—this is where life has brought us.

Each person will approach the boundary between life and death differently because we have composed our lives differently. Some may believe confidently that they have a visa stamped in their passport for safe passage. Others may be terrified before the unknown. Some may even feel the excitement of a new adventure. I believe the majority of people who face the end of life are drenched with many intense but jumbled emotions and can't identify which of their feelings are most real, if any are, and which deceive. No one, though, can be indifferent as he or she walks through that valley under the shadow of death.

Let me talk first about the emotion of fear, because at some level of our being all of us human beings inevitably experience fear of death. Fear of death is not just an emotional reaction, such as what we feel when the telephone rings in the middle of the night. It's more like a pervasive attitude. Not everyone who enters the world of the dying is *controlled* by an attitude of fear (and it's my belief that none of us has to be); but fear is so much a part of the existential crisis of death that every one of us has to make our way through it, not around it. If we pretend it's not there, we can be overtaken and controlled by fear without even realizing what is happening.

It's natural and even normal to experience fear when death is close. Sometimes, though, fear overwhelms us and runs away with us. Let's begin with that extreme case, because it makes the issues sharp and clear. Looking at the dynamics of extreme fear, we can learn how to help a person who is experiencing fear in any degree as he or she faces the end of life.

When fear takes hold, the person is left with very reduced ways of

13

coping with death. *The person who is controlled by fear is basically limited to two postures before death: despair or denial.* The person may oscillate back and forth between despair and denial, and often does, but fear does not allow other responses. We need to examine this dynamic carefully, because it is the mind-trap that blocks many people from accepting the situation and experiencing hope, peace, love, and integrity when they are dying. When fear is in control, picture that shifting between denial and despair to look like this:

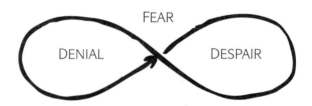

First, think about *denial.* Denial is called a defense mechanism, and so it is—a way of defending ourselves against the fear; a conspiracy, often with loved ones, to keep it unconscious. Denial is a mind-trick that blocks information too threatening to cope with.

When I served as a hospital chaplain, I noticed people using various forms of denial to avoid facing their true conditions. One form, for example, is the "rose-colored glasses" response. The patient will say something like, "Oh, Doctor [or reverend, nurse, family member, or friend], I'm so glad my hemoglobin is looking better this morning! I just know I'm getting better every day!" Now on the face of it, we caregivers usually welcome optimism—we welcome a positive attitude and enter into the conspiracy, even when we recognize it as denial—because it lets us off the hook! The trouble with that patient's response, however, is it blocks out information that gives a whole, truthful picture and lets through only that sliver of information that allows the patient to live in an illusory bubble.

A second form of denial I have heard frequently, maybe because of my role as chaplain, is the "miracle" response. Like optimism, miracle language is not necessarily denial. Caregivers hope and pray for a miraculous cure or remission, sometimes to the very end. Everyone has heard stories of an apparently miraculous recovery. Looking for a miracle becomes denial only when it is used to block out recognition of the whole picture. If the patient says, "I just know God has worked a miracle! The doctors can say what they will, but I'm cured and I'm going home soon," it suggests that someone is using religious notions to avoid reality and to avoid doing the challenging and courageous work of bringing one's life to a close. The *real* miracle of healing at the end of life, I firmly believe, is most often found in this graceful work of seeking reconciliation, completing one's work, and ending one's lifetime.

People use denial only because they have to. When their response to death is motivated primarily by fear, then death is too frightening, too overwhelming, to face, and they avoid the unthinkable by denial. No caring person would brutally knock down that scaffolding and make them fall. They have used precious energy to build it; the scaffold of denial is the only safety they know. To deny a person that defense mechanism would only send them flying over to the only alternative response to death available to them in their fear, which is *despair.*

Despair is to be in the grip of hopelessness and helplessness. The frightful reality of the present moment is all there is, and it can only get worse. One person, a young medical professional dying with cancer of the small intestine, put it in these words: "I fear the loneliness of it all. It's going to get worse; nothing is going to get any better. I'm going down the tube."

No metaphor expresses the terror of hopelessness and helplessness more tellingly than "I'm going down the tube." Such despair numbs the person to feelings and cuts off meaningful communication with loved ones. The sense of being absolutely out of control deprives one of the actions one can take while one has life, such as communicating with loved ones or making a will. Thus the attitude of despair, like denial, stunts life by imposing a kind of emotional and spiritual death on a person who has important work to do and some potentially rich days yet to live.

Trying to help, the caregiver may be tempted to trick the person into believing that things aren't so bad after all—in other words, flipping them over into denial. That may make it easier for the caregiver, but it brings the person no closer to a fully human life and death.

What then can be done to help? If you are a person who has a life-threatening illness, you would not be reading this book if a paralyzing fear of death had driven you into either denial or despair. Maybe the discussion above helps you see traces of those spiritual attitudes (or their psychological counterparts, mania or depression) in yourself, and you will want to address them. I am speaking most directly, though, to caregivers, such as family members, health professionals or pastors, hospice workers, and others. How can we be faithful in accompanying a person through the valley of the shadow of death, so that they may fear no evil, living the days that remain to them with honesty, integrity, and hope? That is the question.

Despair

Begin with the person in the condition of despair . . .

Whenever you face a huge, overwhelming problem, what is the best way to tackle it with any hope of solving it? The answer is common wisdom: you break it down into little problems that, knotted together, make up the huge one. Then, you take on the smaller, simpler problems one by one.

Despair is like an overwhelming problem. A person can't get hold of it—despair is too huge, too powerful, too life-draining. Think of despair within the framework of loss. It is very hard to face the loss of a job, a spouse, a child. When a person faces death, though, he faces the loss of all those things at once and more. That is why it is so overwhelming—the loss is too great to think about. One feels numb before such loss.

As a faithful accompanier you can use that piece of common wisdom, though. You can help the dying person to break despair—global, overwhelming loss, the loss of everything—down into the specific losses that make death grievous for him or her. Then, you can help the person grieve those losses one at a time and find healing.

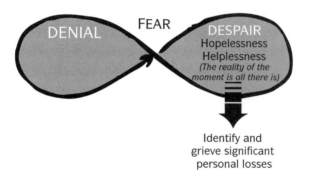

I suggest this with humility and don't want it to sound like a glib solution. A person who faces death may fear annihilation, punishment, or torment, and these existential fears cannot be generalized or taken lightly. There is no one-size-fits-all formula for easing the fears of humankind before death.

And yet, these expressions of personal despair (annihilation, punishment, or torment), are particular ways a human mind has constructed an *interpretation* of death—an event that is in itself natural, neither good nor bad, happening to every living thing. One way to help the person reconstruct his or her personal death, I am suggesting, is to *reframe it in terms of loss*, and then to identify the particular loss or losses that make death fearful and unwanted. Reframing death in terms of loss does not either affirm or contradict the individual's beliefs (or irrational fears). It does, however, bring the matter into the realm of the personal, the relational, where emotions are real and things can be named.

An example may help explain how you can help a person move from paralyzing despair to the ability to grieve losses. The person I mentioned earlier, who expressed his global depression and despair by the dismal image of going down the tube, mentioned in the same conversation that the only time he ever cried was once when he was with his two little children, five and three years old, and realized he wasn't going to be with them much longer. He quickly moved on to talk about something else, but he had dropped a clue that could make the difference in helping him break through his despair. The clue was that one of the things that makes death grievous for him—that contributes to the overwhelming fear that has him in its grip—is the loss of his children, and their loss of him.

I might say to him, "May I ask you about your children?" (When we know we are approaching a sensitive area with emotional risk involved, we ought to ask permission to go there and respect a "no" if it comes.) If he gives permission, I could then ask him to tell me their names, to describe what he loves about each one, which parent they are most like, what he hopes for each of them, how he hopes they will remember him. This conversation will probably be emotional, and could be like pulling out the cork on an emotional life that has been stopped up by fear. The intention is to help him identify specific losses that make his death so terribly saddening, anger-producing, or fearful to him and allow him to *grieve* them.

Grief is not a single emotion. It is a dynamic complex of emotions, including sadness, anger, fear, loneliness, and more, that is triggered by

18

significant loss or the threat of loss. Grieving is remembering, imaging, bringing into one's consciousness the loss, remembering him/her/it in a thousand ways, and feeling the full weight of the emotions contained in each memory until one can progressively *let go of that which can no longer be held onto.* Grieving is the human mechanism for dealing with loss, painful as it is to do so. In fact, healing from the wound of significant loss doesn't happen any other way. Because of that, we can say that grieving is good.

If this man we're speaking of responds to the conversation about his children by opening his heart and allowing emotional energy to flow, one might then, perceptively and sensitively, direct him to identify other losses significant to him. For example, he might feel a sense of loss for his wife, his professional future, his concern for the environment, close friendships, or listening to opera. Gradually one helps him to move from global despair, emotional shutdown, to grieve specific losses by feeling and releasing the sadness, anger, and other emotions packed into them. Note that this approach is very different from trying to deceive him or cheer him up. It *respects* his despair, helping him move to a benign form of it—grieving real losses appropriately. Despair is fear-based, but grief is not.

Something else is beginning to happen. A new spiritual dynamic is becoming possible, which we will name in a moment.

Denial

But first we must look at *denial,* the other fear-based response to death. The principle of intervention is the same: Don't try to knock them out of it because the only place they can go is despair. Instead, respecting their need to protect themselves, inject one or two degrees of reality into your responses. "Mrs. Smith, I'm glad too that your hemoglobin is up today and that you're feeling better," the nurse or doctor might affirm to the person in our earlier example. And then, "I want you to know that if there's a time you are not feeling confident and get worried, or if you feel sicker, you can talk with me about that too. Your illness is still very serious, and we don't think it is getting better."

Such a response: (1) affirms the person where she actually is and reaffirms her need to be there; (2) assures her you are with her in bad news as well as good; (3) makes a distinction between herself and her illness; and (4) lets her know (if she can hear it) that you do not share her expressed sense of what's going on. You're a person she can get real with, when she's ready. Given the conspiracies of denial, you may be the only one.

When persons are in denial, the therapeutic goal is to slip them over to a benign form of denial, which is *the ability to identify with the best possible outcome.* The name of that condition is optimism. There is nothing wrong with optimism, when grounded in reality. A woman I knew well was told by her physician that people in her stage of breast cancer have a 20 percent chance of living for five years. Her response was wonderfully optimistic: "Doctor, with your help and with God's help I intend to be one of those 20 percent! Now tell me what I need to do to make that happen." Using both medical and spiritual resources, she lived for nine more years and, to use her word, she died "healthy."

Was she denying? Well, if she was (and the statistical chances were four to one that she would *not* survive five years) it was a benign form of denial. Why? Because she accepted the realities of the disease, she placed herself in that picture, and she chose to identify with the positive possibility within that picture of reality. In so doing, her positive attitude may have actually increased her chances of achieving the outcome she wanted. That is a very healthy frame of mind, in my view—to identify with the best possible outcome.

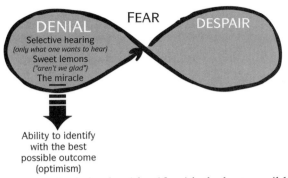

A person can be helped to identify with the best possible outcome, in a framework of reality, by supporting the person's need to think positively without supporting illusion or falseness. Along with this comes the ability to form realistic goals or intentions for the time that remains to him or her. By contrast, a person in denial is paralyzed by fear. *Helping the person move toward more realistic, positive aspirations* (I purposely avoid calling it "hope" at this point) is lessening the hold of fear, and is moving toward the next step, which is hope.

Lance writes . . .

I cannot agree more with Bert's discussion above. From a medical perspective, the role of *denial* in the dying process must receive attention because of its profound influence on the style and quality of care the dying person will eventually receive. As you read the narrative case examples in Chapter 7, the impact of denial will be clear. It may be said that denial is the human tendency to block out painful realities. Our own mortality is often a major point of denial. Most of us do not want to consider our own deaths, or even the deaths of other people. As Bert said, denial can protect us from fear and allow us to function during painful times, but it can also prevent planning and discussing serious issues. When denial blocks our ability to plan, it should be confronted.

Imagine you are terminally ill, and no further treatment will prevent your death in about three months. That is reality. It is painful, but it is the truth. Now, imagine you simply cannot accept that you have only three months to live. You refuse to accept the truth and therefore do not make your plans. You will likely find yourself running fearfully to many doctors and hospitals trying to escape your natural fate. When death does come to the imaginary you who is trapped in denial, how frightening and unpredictable it would be for you and your loved ones. You may have neglected to plan your estate or establish a relationship with a doctor who knows your case well. You may miss a chance to spend time with loved ones. You may miss the chance to appreciate your life and to reflect on its meaning. On a practical note, you will likely miss the chance to actively plan for and manage your own death or to find a trusted companion to assist you with that task. Then you may, unfortunately, find yourself in situations where you have little control. Without proper planning, discussion, and documentation, you may find yourself at the mercy of the medical system, which may care for you in ways you would never choose for yourself. Denial, when left unaddressed, can indeed set us up for less than ideal outcomes.

Now imagine the scenario above with a completely different reaction on your part. Let us say that you seek a reasonable second opinion and find that, indeed, there is no real hope for your recovery. Imagine yourself attempting to accept that reality, to release your denial. You would grieve and feel anger. You may pray and talk to family. You may feel a need to find someone to blame. However, the bottom line is that after you experience your normal emotional range, you accept your fate. You have released denial. Now you can plan. Imagine yourself telling your loved ones the news, calmly and reassuringly, even while being sad. Imagine telling them you will need their help and support, but you are going to plan ahead so you do not suffer and can be home as much as possible until the end. Imagine making plans to see people you have not seen for years and saying "I love you." Imagine taking large chunks of time to teach grandchildren your values and give them the benefit of your wisdom. Imagine showing your children and family that death, while frightening, can be handled with dignity and courage. Imagine knowing that you will not suffer. This is the powerful difference in your reality that can occur if you can allow yourself to release denial.

Now imagine the person dying is not you, it is your elderly, demented mother. Imagine that you deny she is fading, which renders you less able to help her. Alternately, imagine that you accept the fact that her life is closing, and you then take positive and proactive steps to help her through this process with love and support. You can do this. It begins with understanding and acceptance, which progresses to knowledge and action.

Hope

Bert writes . . .

H*ope.* Now we can use the word, as we begin to understand the dynamic integrity it contains. Hope is not the same as optimism. Hope is when the ability to imagine and identify with the best possible outcome is held in dynamic relation with the ability to grieve significant losses appropriately. When the dynamic tension is held and sustained at such a level...that is hope. The completed diagram now looks like this:

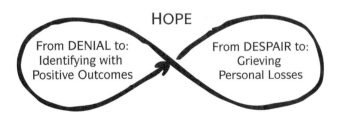

I learned this dynamic of hope from my father-in-law, who was dying of cancer when his grandchildren were still very young. He loved his family above every earthly love and was clearly grieving "not being able to grow up with my grandchildren," as he put it, not continuing to have a part in forming their lives. The rest of the family was also grieving the grandchildren's loss of him. He spent time with them as he was able. And then when Christmas came, someone had the idea of recording the stories he always told that gave the Christmas season such rich and unique coloration in that family. He was a great storyteller, and by using a simple tape recorder his grandchildren could know him that way in later years. Telling the Christmas stories meant so much to him that he went on and recorded all the stories of his Tom Sawyer–like boyhood on a South Carolina farm, stories all his children knew by heart—now his grandchildren could hear those stories too. In other words, grieving his grandchildren helped point to how he could identify with the best possible outcome. He had found a way to "grow up with my grandchildren."

Elisabeth Kubler-Ross pointed out in her groundbreaking book, *On Death and Dying* [1] that hope does not always mean hope for an extended life. More often, in circumstances of terminal illness, it means hope for freedom from pain, hope for reconciliation with an estranged son, hope for dying at home with loved ones present, or hope for a way to continue to be with one's grandchildren. Such hopes are true hopes, because they are possible things (best possible outcomes) held in dynamic relation with a realistic appraisal of losses and grieving those losses. Grieving—yet one identifies and claims positive outcomes. That dialectic, the dynamic of hope, is a healing way into death.

Hope, true hope, allows one to be at rest with the courage to relinquish control, to accept death, to experience peace. *The dynamic of*

---

[1] Elisabeth Kubler-Ross, *On Death and Dying* (Touchstone, 1997, copyright 1969).

hope—between appropriately grieving losses and identifying with the best possible outcome—takes the place of the dynamic of fear. Fear oscillates between denial and despair and diminishes life. Hope can replace fear as the spring or origin of one's response to death. Hope is an attitude that supports full emotional and spiritual living. That is the goal of faithful accompaniment of the dying.

We have seen how hope is a dynamic process that, in a sense, does two opposing things at the same time and keeps them related to each other. Now let's develop that model one step further. First, though, let me tell you about Mrs. Clark, who became a friend of mine.

Once when I was serving as hospital chaplain for my church, I went to see a woman who came into the hospital because of her advanced stage of congestive heart failure. I learned that Mrs. Clark lived alone in a house she and her husband had built on a river far from town. She had been a widow for twenty years, had no children, and her Scottish brogue told me she might not have other family in this country. In fact, I was the only visitor she had.

I saw Mrs. Clark almost daily for the two weeks she was in the hospital. Nothing in her jovial manner or her habits suggested depression, and her readiness to disclose her poor prognosis proved she was not denying anything. Whatever fear she felt of death was not overwhelming her; in fact, she took some Scottish pride in her ability to "look death in the eye." I liked her. Yet, when I was with her, I noticed a kind of wistfulness, a sadness, that seemed to underlie her humor and her general acceptance of her frail condition. I wondered if she was aware of the sadness.

On the third visit, when we were comfortable with each other, I asked Mrs. Clark if she would tell me if there was anything in her life she regretted or that caused her sadness and that might keep her from having a clear conscience. "Yes," she said, "there is. It's something that's been on my mind a lot lately, but there's nothing to be done about it."

Sometimes, I told her, it helps just to say it out loud.

She proceeded to speak of how she was a "blithe young lass" when World War II began. She met an American sailor who was stationed near her town in Scotland. One thing had led to another, and soon she was pregnant. Under severe pressure from her father, she and the sailor were married, not in the church but in the council office. The baby, born several months later, lived only one day. After the war her young husband came back and took her to the United States to live. They had no more children. He went into the timber business, he never expressed his feelings, and she felt he resented her at first, but they became better companions when she learned to share his passion for fishing. No, she did not feel punished when the baby died, just a sadness that never went away, and a feeling that the marriage was false from the start. She was lonely in that marriage.

She told me she had not spoken these thoughts out loud for fifty years, but she had lived with them every day. She expressed shame, anger, and regret. I listened to her tell her personal truth. It felt like a strain, and then release. As a pastor, I received her story and prayed with her, declaring that she was—in spite of it all—uniquely valuable, loved, and accepted.

Then I told her she had dropped hints of what a rich and varied life she'd had, both in Scotland and over here. I asked her to tell me other stories, beginning with her childhood. She told stories for over a week of visits, and I enjoyed them all. Some of the stories related to fishing with her husband, and in them she began to express not just resignation to a lonely marriage but warmth and joy in him as a person. She told of incidents that showed he really did care for her, and I told her I thought maybe she saw that too. A marriage that had seemed, in her earlier confession, empty and false, began to take on other dimensions. Friends came and departed in her stories, as did her career as a country teacher, and her life developed texture. One of the last times I saw her, she said, "I wish you could come see me at the fish camp. It's been a good life there, and I'm satisfied."

Think about that story with me, in light of the hope diagram we discussed earlier. Begin with the *grieving losses* side of the diagram. In my experience as a pastor, I have found that a particular kind of grieving is frequently a key element in a person's finding peace at the end of life. The grieving I speak of is commonly called *confession*. This term may be more frequently used in Roman Catholic than other spiritual traditions, but it refers to an action that's essential to everybody, even the non-religious, in bringing their lifetimes to a close. The caregiver might ask a woman who is dying, "Is there anything you have done, or left undone, that continues to burden your conscience?" The question may be phrased differently to help the person speak of something in her life that she has not been able to release. "Is there anything in your life that you sincerely regret? Is there anyone you've harmed, maybe secretly, from whom you would want to ask forgiveness?"

Just to voice such regrets or harms and express sorrow for them is a release. If the caretaker can assure the person that she is forgiven, or perhaps arrange a direct meeting with the other person affected so forgiveness may be granted by the one harmed, that brings confession to a deeper level of completeness. A still deeper level is when you ask the dying person if she is carrying any grudges—unforgiven harms done to her by another—and then encourage her to forgive that person and let go of the bitter memory. Receiving and giving forgiveness for hurts that have festered, sometimes for most of a lifetime, can possibly be the form of grieving that goes farthest in releasing emotions that encase the heart and keep one from finding peace.

The other side of this spiritual equation, in the dialectic of hope, corresponds to identifying with the best possible outcome. We may call it simply *affirming one's life as it is.* Erik Erikson's best-known contribution to psychology is his description of seven developmental stages of the human journey, each with a task the individual has to perform to be able to move on. The last stage and task of life he called *ego integration*. At the end of life, a person's task is to gather together the many strands of his life and to experience the wholeness of his lifetime. Sometimes the process is called life review. It often consists of telling stories, the stories of a lifetime, and sewing the little stories into a whole story like a beautiful patchwork quilt.

When someone listens, that is affirming. It can be as natural as a grandparent telling stories to a grandchild. Or it can be as structured as a caregiver asking the person to tell about the first day at school, or the wedding day, or first job, or best vacation, or proudest moment. Telling stories helps the person at the end of his or her lifetime to say, with genuine feeling, "This is my life. I didn't accomplish everything I dreamed of, but I'm proud of what I did accomplish. I made some mistakes and I had some successes. But this is my life as I lived it, and I declare that it was good." I think ego integration is always accompanied by an attitude of thanks.

That, I believe, is an honest pathway to *accepting*. Look back a moment. We started with fear, because it is very natural to feel fear when we are close to death. When fear controls us, though, it shuts us down—we can only experience despair or denial. But if someone can help the person facing death to grieve specific losses *and* to identify with the best possible outcome, then that person has found a way to move from fear to *hope*. By the same token, if the helper can allow the person to confess failures and feel forgiveness, and to remember (re-member) and affirm his life, then the person is well on the way to peaceful acceptance.

If anyone would be a genuine companion and helper to a person who is dying, the helper must be free enough, and freeing enough, to accompany at this level of humanness. Otherwise, for example, you have no ability to discern whether the patient's use of a religious

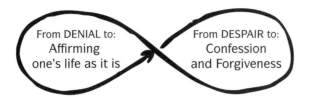

From DENIAL to:
Affirming
one's life as it is

From DESPAIR to:
Confession
and Forgiveness

symbol or doctrine is a source of authentic hope or merely a screen for denial, for it can be either; you may not have the courage needed to cause a person the pain of remembering deep losses so that he or she can grieve them and find release, for it takes great courage to trust human resilience that far. There are no easy formulas, second-hand solutions, pre-fabricated faith responses—they ring false at this level of experience.

What is required to be a faithful companion is love. Courageous, intelligent love. Not facile love, and certainly not love of oneself in the role of caregiver (which sometimes deceives us into thinking we are loving the one who is dying). No, it takes love that is born in one's own spiritual walk—the caregiver's personal wrestling with meaning, a deep sense of human connection, and sensitivity before the mystery of life and death.

The journey from fear to hope is a journey that is made at a spiritual level. Temporal things, concrete details, are the stuff of the journey, however. How we handle pain, whom we will miss, what metaphors are available to us in thinking about death, who is with us "at the close of day." That is why the journey from fear to hope was described in such concrete terms, even though the shift in attitude from fear to hope belongs to the level of spiritual tectonics.

Spirituality, conceived in terms of meaning, connection, and mystery, appears to relate to all humankind at the core. Even so, the particular pathways and insights of historic, living religious traditions are an invaluable help to many people. They give firmer form and more dense substance to people's quest for meaning, to their community of support, and to their encounter with the divine.

Doctor Shopping

Lance writes . . .

The first principle of *The Active Management of Dying* is "Accept the reality of the situation." The implication here is that one is accepting the futility of further medical or surgical interventions and focusing on comfort measures. It takes a lot of trust to accept a doctor's opinion that one is approaching death and there is nothing left that will meaningfully delay or reverse that process. People who have had long-standing relationships with their doctors tend to come by this trust more easily and therefore accept this reality more easily. However, most people do have doubts. Bert and I would always recommend a reasonable second opinion when one is getting news of a terminal disease or incurable condition. A third opinion is also reasonable.

However, some patients and families may opt for a pattern of "doctor shopping." Doctor shopping implies going to multiple new doctors looking for an answer that is desired rather than one based in reality. Some people will see more than ten different doctors, requesting a complete evaluation and treatment. Understandably, these folks want someone to tell them that a cure exists, even when the truth of terminal status is obvious.

The problem with doctor-shopping is that it adds chaos to an already chaotic time. It wastes time that should be spent planning and dealing with grief and relationships. Too many medical opinions can be very confusing, and the provision of comfort care may be delayed far too long.

A reasonable and productive second opinion would include a thorough physical exam and review of the existing studies, such as x-rays, scans, labs, and biopsy results. The second opinion provider may want to repeat certain tests or order new ones. If the second opinion differs significantly from the first, a discussion should center on why the second doctor sees the case differently and what that might mean for the patient. If there is a significant disagreement, a third opinion may be helpful in determining the next step. If the two opinions agree closely, it is very unlikely that further opinions would be very different.

In general, I would have a lot of trust in a doctor who gave an opinion about a serious medical issue but who had the wisdom to recommend a second opinion for the patient's confidence. You should not think a doctor lacks confidence or skill because he or she endorses a second opinion. It is a sign of responsible humility.

Sometimes, when a doctor gives a patient bad news and is very honest about it, the patient may focus his or her resulting anger and frustration on the doctor. In this case, the recipient of the bad news must take a step back and realize that the doctor is not creating the disease that is responsible for the bad news. He or she is merely being honest about the seriousness of the disease so that productive steps can then occur. Patients do themselves a disservice if they allow misplaced anger to drive them away from a doctor who delivers unfortunate news in a straightforward and frank manner. That doctor usually will be a good and trustworthy ally.

Anticipatory Grieving

Bert writes . . .

How can we grasp the reality and significance of what family members go through when a loved one is dying? Can we describe the emotional course, wild pathway that it usually is, with enough clarity so that spouse or partner, adult child, or grandchild can make some sense out of what is going on? If you are reading this because someone you love has a life-threatening condition, you can test the thoughts I am going to share with you against the reality of your own experience.

I want to call the pathway *anticipatory grieving.* Later in this book we will talk at length about grief. Grief is our natural human response to loss. We also grieve, however, when there is the threat or *anticipation* of loss. We begin grieving when we first allow ourselves to be conscious of losing this person we love, with whom we are intricately bonded in relationship. To call it by the name *grief* gives insight into what we are going through during this difficult time.

Grief is basically an *anxiety reaction to loss or the threat of loss.* The main "engine" of grief is *love*—when we imagine the person gone, we feel a deep vacancy in our life that causes a flood of emotions, and sometimes they are overwhelming. It's as though we transport ourselves into the future and feel what the absence will be like, and this causes strong feelings of sadness, fear, and possibly anger. Anticipatory grieving is our anxiety letting loose these strong emotions. It is very hard and exhausting inner work.

Something else is occurring that goes beyond the feeling of absence or vacancy. What also happens is that the primordial anxiety of *separation* is brought to the surface. Every significant loss reaches down into our deeply buried and unconscious memories and pulls up our earliest, most pervasive anxiety—separation from mother. When we lose someone now whose presence we depend on for our personal and emotional stability and well-being, or when we anticipate separation from that one, the energy of our anxiety (grieving) comes from the very bedrock of our selfhood, laid there in infancy. It is like an emotional earthquake. The more significant the loss, the stronger the earthquake.

The name of the feeling released by separation anxiety is *fear.*

Your experience may also make you aware of another kind of anxiety besides separation anxiety, and that is *moral* anxiety. All of us have ambiguous feelings even about those who are closest to us. It is completely normal to sometimes get angry or feel some resentment toward those we love the most. And they feel those same feelings toward us. What happens in anticipatory grieving is that these normal, ambiguous feelings become much more threatening than usual, because death makes the stakes much higher.

We usually experience the anxiety as *guilt*. A wife might think, "How could I be angry with my husband for dying and leaving me alone?" Or an adult child might think, "What kind of person am I to resent having to spend all this time taking care of my dear mother, who sacrificed to take care of me?" Feelings of guilt are a normal part of grieving, and they are most potent before the person has died.

Anticipatory grieving is intensely hard emotional work because we are dealing with anxiety that comes from the very foundations of our selfhood. Both separation anxiety and moral anxiety are inevitable—the threat of loss is like a trigger. If we understand that, we can be more accepting of our feelings and not think we are crazy or bad. It helps to talk about those feelings with another person who can listen carefully to us. Bringing them out into the light may help us recognize the anxiety as coming more from our inner condition than from outer reality.

Yet there is still another factor that makes anticipatory grieving difficult. That is the fact that we are, in a sense, doing two fundamentally opposite things at the same time.

On the one hand we are *letting go*—allowing ourselves to begin grieving the loss even before the loss has occurred, preparing ourselves for the emotional blow we know will come when the death actually happens. In anticipatory grieving, we begin rehearsing in our minds what it will be like to be bereaved—to be in the role of widow or widower, to be without a parent, to live without a child. These thoughts and feelings help us gently to begin the process of letting the loved one go.

On the other hand we are *holding on*. We are not surrendering yet! There is hope still, and we feel we need to muster every ounce of strength and positive thought to help our loved one through. "Giving in" to any acceptance of death while a husband is alive may even cause us to feel *guilty*, as if we are letting him down when he needs us the most to be strong.

What a tension—no wonder anticipatory grieving is such hard work! I don't know any easy way to release ourselves from this tension of beginning to let go at the same time we are trying to hold on. Both are movements of the soul, and both are perfectly normal and understandable.

What we can do, however, is this. We can *give ourselves permission* to gradually allow the letting go to displace the holding on. At the beginning of the illness, especially during the period of aggressive treatment, our thoughts and prayers to strengthen the loved one predominate over our letting go (although "letting go" thoughts will certainly come in unbidden). We are mainly holding on. Later in the illness, after aggressive treatment has been discontinued, we can be more comfortable about consciously letting go and see grieving as appropriate.

All that we have said earlier about how the patient can replace the dynamic of fear with the dynamic of hope (in which she holds grieving the loss of her life in one hand and a desire for the best possible outcome in the other) is true also for those who accompany the dying person. Grieving is thus part of hope, and the grieving part usually accelerates toward the end because death has already begun to be felt in the room. Our need to hold on is now lessened.

When a person grieves in this manner, it can equip him or her to cope better emotionally when the death occurs. The grieving is not finished, of course; the pathway of mourning stretches on ahead, after death, but some of the tasks of normal grieving have already been accomplished. Anticipatory grieving prepares us so that when our loved one's death does occur, we are already familiar with the country of the bereaved and can travel the path of grief that leads through it more effectively and perhaps with less pain.

One common problem in anticipatory grieving lies in the pacing or timing, which is not altogether under our control. I have said that *letting go* gradually replaces *holding on*, so that when death occurs the loved one is better prepared. If anticipatory grieving is foreshortened by a death that comes earlier than expected, that will not have happened. But it is the opposite case that deserves our most careful attention. If the death is delayed, *emotional burnout* can occur. A family can go as far as they can go with anticipatory grieving and the loved one is still there. Let me tell a story to illustrate what I mean.

Some years ago, a 42-year-old woman on the nursing staff of our hospital was diagnosed with stage 4 cervical cancer. She had a very caring husband and four devoted children ranging in age from ten to nineteen. When the cancer was announced it was an immense shock to the family, but they rallied around their wife and mother. When she could go home, they rented a hospital bed and placed it in the living room at the foot of the stairs. The family wanted to surround her with their love during her last days with them. She was at the center of every family activity; one could not come in the front door or move around the house without passing her bed. The family was a model of emotionally open, honest anticipatory grieving. I was in awe of their courage.

But the mother did not die. Month after month she continued to live, the focus of intense emotions, requiring constant care. The family began to unravel. The social lives of the teenagers were totally disrupted and one of them got into serious trouble. Grades dropped. The father began staying at work later and later and separating from the family. What was going on? They had simply burned out emotionally because they could not sustain their grieving to the end. I doubt if they could understand the guilt they felt for feeling angry, frustrated, and unloving toward her, even sometimes wishing she would die.

The health professionals caring for the patient were slow to recognize what was happening, probably because the family had been held up as a shining example of "how to do it." When we did finally see it, the doctor quickly persuaded the husband to let his wife finish her days in the hospital. The husband seemed very relieved when the bed was removed from the living room. Family therapy was offered to help a family that had been heroic in their initial response to a tragic situation but were nearly defeated by its prolongation.

That is the most dramatic case I have witnessed of dysfunctional anticipatory grieving. The intense pressure of the family's grieving could have been lessened by removing the patient from the focal center of the home sooner. If she were in a hospital or hospice facility, or even if she were at home with more alert professional guidance, family members could have "regulated" their active grieving according to their needs—thinking of the metaphor of the thermostat. We do that: we naturally pace ourselves according to our emotional capacity and needs, so that we can go the distance with our loved ones, and then let them go when we can accompany them no longer.

Such a strong negative example can bring to light feelings or problems that other grieving people have to a lesser degree. Issues like these do come up in accompanying a loved one who is dying, and they can usually be resolved. Hospice care provides effective guidance. The main point is that anticipatory grieving is natural and serves a good purpose. Yes, it is difficult, because loss is difficult and because timing is uncertain. By being alert to the dangers—such as ambiguous feelings stabbing us with guilt or distressed caregivers acting out conflicting emotions in damaging ways—we have a better chance of avoiding the dangers. And we can allow the healing properties of grief to make us more ready to "let go" when the time comes. For that is what grief does, and that is why grief is necessary and good—it helps us to let go of one whose physical presence we can no longer keep, and then we can become whole again.

I learned a lot as I read Bert's words on anticipatory grieving. The term sums up a process which I had seen occur many times but never knew what to call it. It is worthwhile to note that in this section he used a case in which the family had to be persuaded to allow the dying person to receive care in an institution rather than at home. In many other instances we describe how families came to terms with taking a loved one home from an institution. This illustrates the concept that each situation is different, but the value of communication, planning, and expert assistance is universal.

Notes

2

Identify *the* Decision-Makers

Bert writes...

There are important decisions to make in end-of-life care, and we will discuss these decisions in detail. The first question to ask, though, is this: *Who is the leader in making these decisions?* How do we identify or name the leader among all the people involved, and where does the buck stop in decision-making?

The short and true answer to that question is this: *The patient is the leader.* The person receiving the medical care is the person, legally and morally, who should be in charge. A competent adult has the right to control what is done to him or her, medically or otherwise. That person may listen to family or other counselors, or even authorize someone else to make the decisions, but theirs is the choice to do so. Morally, that is called the principle of *autonomy.* Autonomy simply means that in terms of human relations, including medical care, each of us is in charge of himself or herself.

Before we proceed to show how autonomy is spelled out in medical decision-making, though, we must point out that autonomy is not absolute in the case of a patient who is seriously ill. The patient should normally be considered the leader in making personal decisions, but that means others are involved too, in different ways and degrees, and sometimes one of them may become the leader. As we talk about the autonomy or leadership of the person who has the illness under various circumstances, think about the appropriate roles of the doctor, other professional staff, courts, spouse or next of kin, family, and friends.

Informed Consent

Autonomy is spelled out medically in the doctrine of *informed consent*. The patient possesses the right and responsibility to consent to (or question or refuse) what the doctor is recommending be done. No one should do anything to you that you don't want them to do. But, on the other hand, the patient does not possess the right to demand or compel the doctor to do things the doctor believes are wrong. Informed consent does not mean "calling the shots." It implies a kind of dance that looks like this: The doctor tries to communicate to the patient all the information she might need to share meaningfully in the decision they must make together, normally including a recommendation or guidance based on medical judgment. And then the patient, with her own interests, values, and concepts of well-being that go beyond just medical benefit, agrees (consents) to the recommendation or negotiates with her doctor for another course of treatment.

Information the doctor should communicate includes the following:

- **The patient's condition.** The doctor should check for realistic understanding by the patient of the information communicated to her, such as by asking her to restate it in her own words.

- **Possible and desirable medical outcomes.** The doctor should find out what the patient considers most desirable within the field of the possible.

- **Recommended procedures for the optimum outcome.** This is what the physician thinks is the best thing to do medically and recommends to the patient.

- **The reasons behind the recommended procedures.** The doctor can think out loud in terms of the risks and benefits of the procedure so the patient can see how the medical judgment is being made.

- **Alternate procedures.** These can also be mentioned, along with their risks and benefits.

All those things may seem complicated, but every step of that process is really necessary for the patient to participate as a full partner in medical decision-making. Adequately informed, the patient can give consent to what the doctor is recommending, which is what usually happens, or the patient can refuse that course of treatment and choose another. Either way, the patient is exercising her right and responsibility to decide upon and authorize what is done to her medically. That is what informed consent is all about. While it may seem as if the physician is leading, what ought really be happening is that the doctor is using professional knowledge—diagnosis, best treatments, and prognosis—to help the patient use her authority to make a wise decision concerning her medical care.

Informed Consent Requires Capacity

Sometimes there is a problem with carrying out the procedures outlined above. The most common problem is when the patient lacks the capacity, mentally or emotionally, to participate fully in the process. Capacity is not the same as "competence" or "incompetence." Incompetence is a legal term. It can only be determined by a court and has to do with declaring a person's inability to exercise legal rights in regard to themselves or their property. The ability or inability to share appropriately in medical decision-making—usually called capacity —is normally determined by the medical staff. They assume that people possess capacity unless there is some compelling reason to doubt it. If there is, they carefully evaluate the patient to determine the limits of the patient's ability to make decisions and communicate them.

A case example will show how this is not always an easy determination to make. Kathryn M., a seventy-year-old retired schoolteacher, had been treated for a year for lymphoma. She had a history of moderate depression since the death of her husband four years previously. Over the last several months she had missed three medical appointments, and her son and his family observed that she was more withdrawn from them. She was admitted to the hospital with fever, a low white blood cell count, and a possible diagnosis of septicemia. Her physician told her the condition was life-threatening and recommended a course of antibiotic therapy that would likely make her well. She refused the therapy.

Kathryn's understanding of her condition and the recommended treatment was adequate, and she knew the disease would probably end her life if it was not treated. She stated she was ready to die if that was the outcome. On the face of it, therefore, the doctor had warrant to respect her decision to refuse treatment, and that would be the end of the matter. The doctor wondered, though, to what extent her depression was affecting her decision. He knew that a depressed person may have capacity for clear thinking and the expression of those thoughts, but have altered decision-making capacity owing to the darkness in mood or outlook. Would the patient be choosing differently if the depression could be helped first? Should he treat her with the antibiotic while also helping her with the depression? Should her son be brought into the decision-making process, and if so, how? By exerting pressure on his mother to change her mind, or by overriding her decision and becoming her surrogate decision-maker? Would that even be possible legally?

That is an example of how some coercive factors such as depression, early stages of dementia, drug effects on the brain, intoxication, or other internal or external pressures can enter the picture and raise the question of capacity: Is this person choosing freely and rationally?

In the case I have given, a consulting psychiatrist could help by making an evaluation and recommendation concerning the patient's depression. Her pastor could help by assessing her spiritual reasoning in regard to her expression of readiness to die instead of choosing a longer life. It must be determined whether her refusal of life-prolonging treatment is a valid decision by a capable adult possessing the right to choose something others may believe is not in her best interest, or whether she is compromised by the internal coercion of depression, in which case someone else should decide for her. Borderline cases like this one require careful evaluation and unbiased judgment. Consultants (a psychiatrist and pastor in this case) and hospital ethics committees can help.

Some cases of incapacity are much more obvious. When a patient is unconscious or in a coma, has significant dementia or some incapacitating form of mental illness, or is legally incompetent, decision-making authority passes to a legal guardian (if there is one) or next of kin. Some states have laws that rank "next of kin" to avoid confusion and conflict in determining who the surrogate decision-maker should be. Lacking that guidance, it is usually common sense that determines who the surrogate leader is. All states authorize surrogate decision-making for patients who clearly lack capacity or are otherwise declared incompetent.

Advance Directives

Health Care Power of Attorney

Many people think it wise to prevent any ambiguity or confusion as to who their surrogate decision-maker should be. They file what is called a *health care power of attorney* (HCPOA), also known as a *durable power of attorney for health care.* Official forms for all the states that have them are provided free on the Internet at **www.atthecloseofday.com** where you can easily find one. Although some people choose to consult an attorney, this is not required. Generally, notarization is all that is needed to make end-of-life documents legal.

The HCPOA is a "springing" power of attorney that only goes into effect if and when you become incapacitated; otherwise, you remain in control. If you do become incapacitated, the person you have named is authorized to give informed consent or refusal for you. If you name such a surrogate with HCPOA, you should carefully instruct that person as to what your preferences are concerning end-of-life care, and how you want the surrogate to act for you if some specific things should happen to you.

Living Will

This instruction can be done in large part by enacting a second kind of directive, the *living will.* In our state, the official or statute form of this document is named the "Declaration of Desire for a Natural Death." The forms differ from state to state; but free, state-specific copies may be found on the Internet at **www.atthecloseofday.com**.

The living will, also called a *Declaration,* like the HCPOA, can be enacted by a healthy person as a precaution for the future, or by someone going into the hospital for treatment, or as one enters a retirement community or nursing facility. The sooner the better, we say. Make multiple copies and give them to family members, physician, clergy, and attorney. That is, do not put your living will away where nobody can find it in an emergency. It should be accessible. The directives only become valid, however, after a patient is declared by at least two physicians to be terminally ill.

The general intent of the living will is to prevent unwanted efforts to keep you alive with technology after the point that your body can no longer sustain life and will never be able to do so again. Many jurisdictions also make provision for you to declare that you would choose not to be kept alive if you were diagnosed as being in a persistent vegetative state. That is a state in which an individual's capacity for consciousness or awareness is lost permanently because of brain damage, but the parts of the brain mainly in the spinal column are able to keep the heartbeat, breathing, and other vital functions going, sometimes for years.

You may (and should) speak informally with physicians and family members about how you wish to be treated if you should be terminally ill and unable to speak for yourself. And those verbal advance directives should be honored, ethically speaking. If you fill out a living will, however, it makes that conversation more formal and precise and gives it the force of law.

The living will, or Declaration, and the HCPOA can both be used together to assure the highest level of personal responsibility in making decisions at the end of life.

Out-of-Hospital/EMS DNR Order

Lance writes...

The patient and family have the responsibility to complete the health care power of attorney and the living will. The physician then has the responsibility for writing orders that protect the patient from unwanted interventions. The "Do Not Resuscitate" (DNR) order written in the hospital chart tells the hospital staff that no resuscitative measures (CPR, breathing tubes, electrical shocks) are to be administered as the patient dies naturally.

However, if the patient leaves the hospital with an end-of-life plan, a second form of Do Not Resuscitate order must be signed by the physician to prevent emergency medical service (EMS) personnel from performing those unwanted interventions if the patient stops breathing or the heart stops pumping during transport to or from the home or institution. This order is a state-specific document that goes by a variety of names, such as the EMS DNR, the Bedside DNR, and the Out-of-Hospital DNR. Even though it seems redundant and even annoying to add another document to a complex care plan, this document is crucial. Although the physician must sign it, I would advise the patient and family to be sure to ask about it.

Because each state has a different policy regarding out-of-hospital resuscitation by EMS, the details are beyond the scope of this book. Many doctors are not fully aware of this document either and may not have them in the office. However, in order to help you with this additional step we have done research on each state's policy. Initial information is provided at **www.atthecloseofday.com** under "Out-of-Hospital DNR by State." We were amazed by the differences between states and the complexity of some of the policies, but we tried to give you some details and some contact information. We will work to keep the site updated for your convenience.

The Role of the Surrogate

Bert writes . . .

When you are the leader and making surrogate decisions for an incapacitated patient, the binding principle governing your actions is always to decide as you believe the patient himself would decide if he were capable. This ethical principle is called *substituted judgment.* This is true whether you, as a surrogate, are acting formally with power of attorney or informally as next of kin. Ask this question: What would the patient be choosing in this situation, in view of his own interests and values? More than likely, this will be in accord with what you think is the best interest of the patient, but that may not always be the case. Keep in mind that you are acting as surrogate because you are presumed to know the patient best and know what he wants and feels and believes. Put yourself in his place, as much as you can, when you decide on his behalf.

The principle of *substituted judgment*—the surrogate choosing what he believes the patient would be choosing—gives direction in that difficult situation when an elderly parent, now incapable of decision-making, has several children, and they cannot agree on care. If one of the children has spent more time with the parent, living close by or even being the caretaker for a time, that individual may be presumed to know best the wishes of the parent concerning end-of-life decisions. The one who knows best the mind of the patient should be the leader.

The obvious exception to the rule of substituted judgment is when parents make decisions for their child who is a minor. They act purely for what they believe is best for their child.

How the Process Works

In the example I cited at the beginning of this chapter, how could the case play out to show us how this business of patient leadership and surrogate decision-making works? Here's a possible scenario:

Recall that the patient, Kathryn M., is a seventy-year-old woman with lymphoma who is refusing recommended treatment for a life-threatening infection. There are grounds to believe her refusal is possibly due to depression. Let's say that both the psychiatrist and the pastor are consulted by the patient's physician. The consult psychiatrist examines the patient's record and interviews her in the hospital. The psychiatrist believes the patient is oriented and rational but impaired by a clinical depression. He recommends a change of medication and believes the new prescription might relieve the depression, with continued therapy by a social worker or other counselor. The pastor, who has known the patient since before her retirement and her husband's death, believes that her hopelessness does not reflect a peaceful acceptance of death so much as unresolved grief from the loss of her husband and her retirement from teaching, where she had previously felt useful. He believes that both can be helped. Her son agrees.

The hospital ethics consultant, who has this information, questions the son further about his mother's attitude toward life before her depression. He asks if she ever expressed any feelings or stated any preferences about her lymphoma and medical treatments. Her son, also a schoolteacher, describes his mother as a woman who is sensitive, introverted, much loved by her students (and by her grandchildren), a "natural teacher" who invested herself fully in her vocation, and who was deeply at a loss when she retired and her husband of forty-five years died, both of which occurred within a space of two years. She had given no advance directives and never spoke of death. He knows she loves people and life itself. And he believes the family can help her see she is not a burden, and that she can reinvest in living, if her medical condition allows it. The doctor had told him there was a good chance his mother would respond to the antibiotic therapy.

The hospital ethics consultant then advises the attending physician to write Kathryn's initial refusal of treatment into her medical record, along with the report from the psychiatrist and that of the pastor and the remarks of her son. He proposes that, with her son's consent, she be given antibiotic treatment for her medical condition while at the same time her depression is being treated and she is receiving the support of family and church. The physician brings this plan to her and she accedes to it ("assent" is different from full consent) with a sigh of resignation. That is enough. The son's consent is taken as necessary and sufficient because of the diagnosis of clinical depression, supported by the testimony of the pastor and the family.

After two weeks of treatment, the bacterial toxins in her blood are reduced, and she is dismissed from the hospital. Her mood disorder has lifted somewhat, perhaps owing to the change of medication, the attention of her family, and the support from her church. At the next visit her physician draws her attention to the availability of advance directives. She talks them over with her son and fills out both, naming him as her HCPOA. They agree further that if her cancer gets worse and can no longer be treated, hospice care would be appropriate, because she is sure she does not want any extraordinary measures to keep her alive, and she never wants to be a burden to her son and his family. At her request, her son checks out several hospice options in her city.

Summary of the Process

Not all cases in which a patient's full autonomy is compromised by some coercive factor will play out exactly like this. Still, the illustration shows the main features of the informed consent process when it's complicated by doubt as to the patient's capacity. Here is a summary of the salient points in the process:

- An adult, competent person has the right to determine what is done to him medically. This is known as the principle of autonomy. That person is normally the leader in decision-making.

- The patient can extend his right and responsibility for self-determination beyond the point he might become incapacitated. This is done by making an advance directive, such as the living will and/or the health care power of attorney (HCPOA).

- When someone becomes incapacitated, a surrogate (usually the patient's next of kin unless someone else has been formally appointed) is authorized to stand in for the patient in the medical decision-making process. That person becomes the leader for decisions.

- The physician has the obligation to inform the patient (or surrogate) of his medical condition, what medical treatment is recommended, the reasoning behind this recommendation, including the likelihood of attaining medical goals with and without the treatment, and what reasonable alternatives exist to the recommended treatment.

- The patient (or surrogate) authorizes treatment by consenting and communicating consent to the physician. The patient may also refuse the treatment or negotiate another. If it is not possible to reach agreement, the patient may change doctors.

- The whole process should flow in such a way as to respect the personhood and leadership of the patient and employ the professional knowledge and skill of the physician to bring about the best outcome possible.

Moral Decision-Making

Making necessary decisions wisely about medical care at the end of life is both possible and absolutely important. Some of the decisions that lie in our paths cause us to draw deeply from the values and principles that guide our lives. These decisions are *moral* decisions because they tap into beliefs about what is good and bad, or right and wrong, and because they are shaped by the qualities of selfhood that have given us character as persons. These qualities might include courage, honesty, fairness, mercy, and loyalty, to name several that many of us hope we are building into our lives. Moral decisions are choices that rest on those kinds of beliefs and personal qualities.

And these decisions are moral *decisions* because something makes our choice conflicting. We must choose this and let go of that, while there may be some good or bad on both sides. When persons choose to enroll in hospice, for example, they are choosing a pathway of physical, spiritual, and family support that offers a peaceful and dignified experience at the end of life. But they are letting go a more aggressive, hospital-based treatment course that could possibly extend their lives by days or weeks. There are pluses and minuses for them on both sides, but they choose one and let go the other. Moral decisions are choices that force us to affirm one course of action and "cut off" (the original meaning of the word "decide") the others.

How do we make moral decisions in end-of-life care? We do so out of a mixture of subjectivity and objectivity.

Objective Factors

Consider the objective factors first. I will name three:

1. **Law.** This is something that applies to everybody equally. Some matters are decided by legislatures and are called statute law. An example of statute law is the enactment by state legislatures of "natural death acts" that provide for what is popularly called the living will. Other matters are decided by courts when they rule on a particular case. Such case law, which spells out arguments specific to a single case, has strong weight in stating the principles and forming the legal climate in which medicine is practiced far beyond the jurisdiction of the particular court that makes the ruling.

2. **Moral consensus.** This is more difficult to define but just as real when it exists. Examples of moral consensus include the acceptability of physicians giving an analgesic (pain-killer) to a dying patient when it is necessary to still the pain, even if the medicine

may also result in shortening the patient's life. Perhaps there is a doctor somewhere who would not agree to do this, but the vast majority agree to it and know they will not be prosecuted legally for doing so. It is "standard medical practice." General agreement about certain practices by practitioners gives a measure of objectivity to decision-making.

3. **Conscience.** This is the most difficult factor to defend as an objective feature of decision-making because each person's conscience is unique. I am speaking, though, of the belief that there is a natural law, or a revealed truth, that defines actions as right or wrong. Many people believe there are rules, commandments, rights, or obligations that are given and that ought to be followed when they make decisions. That belief gives their decision-making a more objective cast. The decision becomes more a process of discovery and application than of constructing a judgment about what is best under the circumstances. The authority of these pre-existing rules or commandments usually derives from a religious or philosophical commitment.

Subjective Factors

The subjective side of decision-making has to do with the personal judgments we make from our values and principles and personal character, without appeal to any other authority. Even when there are objective factors in our decision-making, such as a law, there is still discretionary space in which we bring our own views and values to the front and choose amidst the uncertainty. For people whose consciences do not contain a large number of pre-existing "oughts," that subjective space will be larger than for those who do believe in natural or revealed laws. But no one is exempt from the risk and freedom of choosing and taking responsibility for their choices.

Let me give an example of what I have just said. A person who holds to a belief in the sanctity of life and/or the commandment "Thou shalt not kill" is likely to exclude some forms of physician-assisted dying that another person, who thinks in terms of supporting quality of life (a subjective valuation), would not exclude. Even so, the first, rules-oriented person must use discernment in marginal instances, such as determining whether withholding force-feeding through a stomach tube (allowing the patient to die) is or is not "killing," or does in fact violate the principle of sanctity of life.

Obtaining Help

Fortunately, one person certainly can *help* another in making those difficult choices. In the pages that follow, we will try to help by bringing some logical structure into ethical issues that are very common in end-of-life medical care. We won't and can't tell anyone what they ought to do or what the "right" decision is. By framing the issues, however, and pointing out where law or consensus exists, we may be able to help you call on your own values to make wise and accurate choices.

Two questions will guide our discussion of moral or ethical issues. What happens when further treatment is ineffective? And how far should doctors go in assisting one to die? These questions really belong to a larger one: What is the ultimate goal of care? This will be the subject of the next chapter.

Notes

3

Discuss *the* Ultimate Goals *of* Care

Bert writes . . .

What if you have implemented an aggressive treatment plan and you come to a point where it is no longer working? Sometimes the doctor recognizes the treatment is no longer contributing to any medical goals, yet the patient or his family will continue to say "Do everything possible, Doctor!" And sometimes it's the patient or his family who realizes the burden of the treatment is no longer worth any good that could result from it and asks that it be stopped, but the medical staff refuses to discontinue treatment. It can work either way, and either way results in a major problem.

Part of the problem is how we define and understand "ineffective." When is a treatment ineffective? There is no scientific answer to that question. We know there is always something else that can be done.

Some further step can be taken, or a treatment continued longer, that offers the possibility of some marginal contribution toward some goal, such as extending life. An extreme (and comic) example of that was the film where the old dictator was dying, piece by piece, until his nose was the only part still alive, so his nose was being kept on life-support systems. When do you say "enough"? When do you draw the line on aggressive treatment and make the transition to palliative (comfort) care?

Start with Attitudes

Where people draw the line on aggressive treatment is a function of their attitudes toward life and their attitudes toward death. This applies to doctors as well as patients.

One fairly common attitude is that death is the enemy and should always be fought and resisted to the last. Some doctors see death as defeat and try to keep their patients alive at whatever cost. Some patients feel such fear that they put death off as long as it can be kept away. Some families are unable to let go of a loved one. All of these see death as the enemy and fight it to the end. They might agree with the sentiments of Welsh poet Dylan Thomas, who attended the death of his father. His famous poem, "Do Not Go Gentle Into That Good Night," [2] begins with these lines:

> Do not go gentle into that good night,
> Old age should burn and rave at close of day;
> Rage, rage against the dying of the light.

Thomas wrote those words of rage and resistance before modern life-support systems were invented. I wonder if today he would be a death-postponer, insisting that everything be done to keep his dying

---

[2] Dylan Thomas, *Poems of Dylan Thomas* (New Directions Publishing Corp., 1952).

father alive as long as possible. The attitude that sees death as the ultimate enemy often (but not always) drives a person or professional to draw the line very late in treatment, if they are willing to draw the line at all.

On the other end of the spectrum, some people might be called death-welcomers, at least when they reach the later stages of their illness. This may be the attitude of people interviewed by Elisabeth Kubler-Ross for her influential book, *On Death and Dying*. She described the final stage of the process of terminal illness as "peaceful acceptance," and found that some of us arrive at such an accommodation before we die. My favorite passage expressing this attitude was written by Indian poet Rabindranath Tagore: [3]

> I was not aware of the moment when I first crossed the threshold of this life.
>
> What was the power that made me open out into this vast mystery like a bud in the forest at midnight?
>
> When in the morning I looked upon the light I felt in a moment that I was no stranger in this world, that the inscrutable without name and form had taken me in its arms in the form of my own mother.
>
> Even so, in death the same unknown will appear as ever known to me. And because I love this life, I know I shall love death as well.
>
> The child cries out when from the right breast the mother takes it away, in the very next moment to find in the left one
> its consolation.

Those whose understanding of death is like Tagore's are likely to be perfectly willing to go gentle into that good night. They will draw the

---

[3] D. J. Enright, *The Oxford Book of Death* (Oxford University Press, 1987).

line of transition from aggressive to comfort care earlier in the treatment process. Or, as I have often seen it, a person who is ill may first feel like fighting and resisting with all he's worth, and then gradually come to an attitude of peaceful acceptance. People's attitudes may often change.

Defining Ineffective Treatment

This brings us to the consensual definition of futile treatment or *medical futility*—that is, ineffective treatment. There are really two sides to it.

The first and narrowest definition is the physiological one. Treatment is ineffective and should not be done when it has been ineffective the last hundred times the doctor has tried it in these circumstances. If quantitative research data exist, then one should judge that if a treatment has been shown to work in less than 5 percent, or very conservatively 2 percent, of trials, it should be deemed ineffective and not used. Even if the patient or family demands it, the ethical physician should not initiate or continue medically ineffective treatment. Some states, such as Virginia, have laws that protect physicians from being pressured by patients or families to act against their professional judgment by continuing to do "everything."

The other side of futility/ineffective treatment is patient-centered and qualitative. Treatment is ineffective when the patient or the surrogate weighs the burden of treatment against the benefits and determines that further treatment is undesirable at this point. For example, whether or not the ventilator support is serving a purpose for a patient is really the patient's call (or the surrogate's call, in this case). It may be medically effective in pumping the lungs and extending life, but is that what the patient values now? The patient may declare that ventilator support is not effective in sustaining the kind of life that is of any real value to him; therefore, being ineffective, it should cease.

Any workable definition of ineffective treatment must include both of these sides. The quantitative side is related to medical futility: the treatment has been shown in medical trials to be ineffective under these circumstances. The qualitative side is the patient's or surrogate's judgment that the treatment is no longer helping to achieve or sustain an acceptable quality of life, or is doing more harm than good. The conclusion we should draw from both or either definition is the same: stop the treatment.

The Ultimate Goal of Care

Note well! Stopping aggressive treatment does not mean stopping *all* treatment. It does not mean the patient is now abandoned by the medical team. It does mean, however, that we stop treatment aimed at altering the disease and make a transition to *comfort care*, which does everything possible to support quality of life in all the days, weeks, or years left to the patient. That is a proper goal—perhaps the ultimate goal—of medical care. The wonderful family physician and writer Ferroll Sams said something like this shortly before he retired from his practice in Georgia: "When I first started practicing medicine I thought I was there to save lives. Later I thought I was there to help people live better. Now I think I'm there to help people die."

How Far Should Doctors Go in Assisting Death?

The intuitive reader will know that Dr. Sams did not mean he should go around giving people that little shove into death, like the resolute body-collector in the film *Monty Python and the Holy Grail.* The plague victim's weak plea, "I ain't dead yet!" brought a swift knock on the head! No, Dr. Sams meant that the physician has the humane and merciful role in our culture of enabling a person to experience dying with dignity and peace.

For physicians, empowering a patient with dignity may mean allowing him to rage against the dying of the light. For another patient it will mean turning off the ventilator, or for another, hearing her request help in foreshortening her life by suicide. How far should doctors go in assisting a patient's dying?

Since that is a question that doctors must ask themselves, I will speak now primarily to the doctor and other caretakers, professional or volunteer, and invite patients to listen in.

G. K. Chesterton said that ethics is like art—you begin by drawing a line somewhere. Here again it's a matter of drawing lines. First, though, let me map out the terrain where a line will have to be drawn. I will do so by listing medical interventions, ranging from something that almost all doctors would be willing to do, to something that most doctors would definitely not do and would be prosecuted for if they did.

A Graded List of Medical Interventions

1. Stopping pain and hastening death. The patient is terminally ill and experiencing intractable pain. The doctor believes that the level and kind of analgesic (pain-killer) required to ease the pain and make the patient comfortable will also depress the respiratory system and probably cause death to come sooner. The doctor explains this, and the patient understands and readily consents. The intention is to stop the pain, and that is the primary effect; the secondary effect is to hasten death.

Some doctors would do this, but then would draw the line and not go further. To them, the rest of the acts listed below imply some intention to foreshorten life, and they believe any act done with that intention is wrong.

60

2. Withholding treatment. The patient is terminally ill and in such a weakened condition that when another system fails, the doctor decides not to begin treating it, possibly because the patient couldn't tolerate the added treatment. For example, the physician withholds dialysis because it would be futile treatment, or does not place the patient on a ventilator, or does not treat pneumonia with antibiotics. Do Not Resuscitate orders also fall into this category: resuscitation is withheld because it could not accomplish any worthwhile medical goal, and the trauma of the attempt would be inhumane.

Some doctors would be willing to withhold treatment when it couldn't be expected to contribute to the ultimate goal of care, but they draw the line here and would not go further to stop treatment. Their reasoning is that it is a more violent act to stop or withdraw treatment already started than never to start it at all. Withholding treatment from the start simply allows nature to take its course, they say—death is less doctor-determined.

3. Withdrawing (stopping) treatment. The patient is terminally ill, and either the treatment being given to keep the patient alive is not working or it no longer seems morally justified to prolong life. The doctor therefore stops the treatment by disconnecting the patient from life-support systems. Our earlier discussion of stopping ineffective medical treatment would usually fit in this category.

Some doctors would readily stop ineffective or unwanted treatment on a dying patient because this too is allowing what we call a natural death—the cause of death is the disease process, the doctor is just getting out of the way. They believe there is no moral difference between withholding and withdrawing treatment. The intention and outcome of both are the same—allowing a dying person to die. Beyond this point, however, the interventions no longer simply allow death but in some degree cause it.

4. Furnishing means of suicide. The patient is terminally ill, and wishes to feel some measure of control by having the means to end his or her own life if the pain or suffering becomes intolerable. The patient asks the doctor for pills, such as sleeping pills, and the information about what dose must be taken to assure a quick and painless death. The patient is willing to promise the doctor to continue the conversation and not use the pills without notifying the doctor first. There may be other stipulations, such as a waiting period before the pills are given (to ensure the patient is not being impulsive), family agreement with the plan, or psychiatric certification that the patient is of sound mind.

Some doctors are willing to grant the patient this measure of control over his or her own life. With the assurance of the patient's full awareness and capability to make such a decision, they honor the person's autonomy by helping the timing of the death. They realize that physician assistance with prescription and information may be necessary for a terminally ill person who is very restricted in movement and could not otherwise secure the means of suicide. They draw the line here, however, unwilling to take a more active role in the death itself.

5. Active euthanasia. The patient is terminally ill, and asks the physician to end his or her suffering by giving a lethal injection or some other means that would cause death. The physician may accede to this request, feeling there is no significant moral difference between putting the means of death in the patient's hands and implementing those means himself, especially if the patient is too impaired to do it.

While a case can be made for the physician implementing the patient's death quickly and mercifully, no consensus exists that the physician's role should be extended this far. In fact, the majority of doctors, including the American Medical Association's Council on Ethical and Judicial Affairs, argue forcefully against it. Their arguments include the following points: Physicians would lose the trust of the public if they were perceived as sometimes healers, sometimes executioners; when the means of death are administered by the doctor, it is less possible for the patient to change his mind at the last minute and stop the process; and physicians would experience an intolerable conflict in their professional mandate to promote health and healing if they were required to be agents of death.

I hope this list of possible interventions will help you discuss and decide how far the doctor should go in assisting the patient in dying. This is an ethical issue that physicians—and policy makers—wrestle with. In the absence of a clear, consensual answer, honest discussion is essential.

Myths about Dying

Lance writes . . .

At this point it seems appropriate to address some commonly held misconceptions about the dying process. It would be unfortunate to let misleading information distract one from the important work ahead. Many myths and misinformation arise from the assumption that the needs of a person who is actively living are the same as the needs of a person who is actively dying. This simply is not true. It is like saying that the needs of an infant are the same as those of an adult.

"Dehydration and starvation are cruel and painful ways to die."

Perhaps the most common misconception is that it is cruel or painful to allow a person to die from dehydration or starvation. This is simply not the case. People tend to use food to nurture and please each other, and most Americans associate initial hunger pangs with the long-term sensations people would feel if they were not fed. However, a tremendous amount of learning and experience on the subject point to the same idea: When a human being reaches the point where he or she cannot or will not accept fluid and food by mouth, he or she is approaching a peaceful passing. If artificial feedings are not initiated through tubes and lines, the person will fall quietly asleep over a period of hours to days. The life processes will slow down gradually, and eventually death will occur. Hunger pangs will pass after the first hours, and the thirst sensation will be diminished markedly by good mouth care (moistening/cleaning).

The exact length of time for death to occur after the withdrawal of water and food will vary by person but usually will be less than one week. This style of death usually will be calm and peaceful, often with no medications required. It is not cruel or painful to the patient, and generally does not cause fear or panic in people who observe it. As long as the mouth is kept moist and comfort medications are available, death can be seen as a pleasant passing.

It is important to be committed to complete withdrawal of fluids and food. Some patients who no longer take in nutrition are given intravenous fluids in an attempt to "ease suffering." This is a mistake and can cause suffering if a person does not receive nutrition. He or she will become depleted of protein and electrolytes. If intravenous fluids are administered to a patient in this state, swelling will occur in the lungs and limbs, causing a drowning sensation and painful skin conditions. Therefore, fluid and nutrition should be withheld simultaneously to help the dying patient avoid suffering.

In recent years we have seen a controversial case in Florida, in which a woman with irreversible brain damage has been and will be in a persistent vegetative state for the rest of her life. Although her husband wanted to withdraw the feeding tubes and allow her to die naturally, her parents objected. The governor of Florida spoke against withdrawal of support and for keeping her alive in a perpetually comatose state. Recently, the

Pope of the Roman Catholic Church, despite some disagreement within the Catholic hierarchy, has taken a similar stance. He announced his belief that there is a moral obligation to continue artificial feedings and hydration in such cases. This edict may profoundly affect the care of many people, especially in Catholic hospitals.

I cannot argue directly with these men or their positions within the context of this book. I know that each is speaking his conscience from his particular perspective. I will simply restate my own experience and training.

I have seen many individuals who are bed-bound and neurologically devastated die naturally once artificial feedings and hydration were withdrawn. It has always been peaceful and relatively swift. On the other hand, I have seen many others kept alive long past their natural lifespans via long-term feeding tubes. Almost always, these individuals demonstrate great pain as their skin inevitably breaks down, infections set in, and muscles wither and contract, despite the best efforts of their caregivers. It is a cruel and nightmarish reality for thousands of people in the U.S. alone. I cannot believe that forcing such a fate on someone is the morally correct course.

I am sure that if either of these leaders were to spend long hours intimately involved in the care of these vulnerable and helpless people, they would gain a different perspective. I assume that each one believes it is better to die of anything else than starvation, but I cannot see how death by pneumonia, sepsis, or heart attack can be considered superior. The important point is that when death is approaching, comfort care is maximized. Each individual involved in end-of-life care may face tough decisions such as these, and I would hate to see guilt and dogma force someone into a decision they would not otherwise make.

*"I will get into legal trouble if I do not call
EMS/911 if someone is dying at home."*

This concern may arise because people are aware of the investigations
that go on regarding elder abuse either at home or in a nursing home.
Caretakers and family members do not want to be accused of neglect-
ing a family member. However, it is very important to understand that
the whole point of *The Active Management of Dying* and good end-of-life
care is that a plan is developed among all people concerned. First, if
the patient has advance directives or cannot speak for herself, and this
is documented, then everyone involved is protected. If the health care
power of attorney makes decisions for comfort care at home, and this
is documented, then again the protection is afforded. If the physician is
involved and makes notes about the plan, then once again the caretaker
is not accused of wrongdoing. If hospice is involved, then it is another
clear sign that the appropriate care is being implemented and neglect
is not an issue. Without some plan documented, recorded, and agreed
upon by the principle members of the plan, however, there is some
risk of inquiry into the cause and manner of death. By following the
basic principles of *The Active Management of Dying,* this potential threat
is neutralized.

Remember that the Out-of-Hospital DNR, in states that have such
a document, is very important in several situations. We are working
to provide free copies of state-specific Out-of-Hospital DNRs on our
website, and they can often be obtained at your local hospital, doctor's
office, or EMS service.

"If someone goes into hospice care,
then they cannot access any further medical care."

While it is true that if a patient enters into the hospice care system, the idea is that they do not make further trips to the emergency room or hospital, this is not an absolute rule. If a hospice patient changes her mind or her surrogate changes his mind, standard medical care can be instituted. It should be stressed again, however, that when one uses hospice care and returns to medical care, once medical futility is certain, one loses much of the benefit that smooth and proper hospice care can offer.

"When someone dies it is always a dramatic scene."

A human being may pass in many different manners. The words "always" or "never" simply do not apply. Depending on the person's constitution, state of health, and reason for dying, the death may be dramatic or peaceful. The goal of proper end-of-life care is to ensure a peaceful death.

"When someone dies it is always a peaceful scene."

See above.

"There is a system set up to
'actively manage' dying people."

Each community has different resources available to assist with the care of the dying. We have offered some information about hospice, and more may be found on the National Hospice and Palliative Care Organization's website, **www.nhpco.org.** In addition, home health nursing, hospitals, doctors' offices, nursing homes, religious institutions, and emergency and social services may all play a role. Unfortunately, there is not a one-stop shop when one is planning the care of the dying. The medical and social service system is very complex, and it does require some study and learning in order to plan the proper care of the dying. It would be unwise to passively depend on "the system." It is much better to work actively with the system. Again, we hope this book will prove a valuable resource as you travel that road.

"All doctors feel the same about the care of the dying."

Doctors are human beings. Each comes from a different background and carries a different set of human values. Physicians do try to follow standards of care and ethical guidelines, but there remains much individual variation in interpretation. Some doctors see the death of any patient as a failure, so therefore will feel obligated to do "everything" for every patient. Other doctors may have a very liberal view of the dying process and will go as far as to euthanize a patient.

An important factor is the stance the patient and the family take when negotiating a plan with the doctor. It is important for the patient and family to view it as a negotiation. When the patient and the family enter the doctor-patient relationship already planning and learning about these issues, perhaps with a living will and HCPOA already completed, the care plan can be more productively addressed. It is vital for the patient and family to find a physician whose values and style match the ideals and desires of the patient.

"Physicians can closely predict a patient's life expectancy."

With enough information, a physician can have a rough idea of a patient's life expectancy. It is based on this that we make referrals to hospice, which generally requires a patient's life expectancy to be less than six months in order to enroll. However, no physician can predict the exact life expectancy for any human being. Each person has a different constitution, a unique will-to-live, and his or her own physical and emotional reserves. It is probably best for the physician to simply make the decision that a patient has reached the dying process and that medical futility has been reached, without trying to pinpoint the exact remaining time. Of note, hospice care has increased its scope in the last several years to include patients with end-stage pulmonary disease (emphysema, chronic bronchitis) on the assumption that these folks reach a point of medical futility with a short life expectancy. However, many of these patients, once they receive the increased attention and care provided in the hospice model, actually improve clinically to the point that they "graduate" from hospice...without any new medical interventions. This example demonstrates that predicting life expectancy cannot be an exact exercise.

Sometimes, when death is very close, the family needs a "best guess" from the doctor so that out-of-town relatives can make plans to be in attendance. In these instances the family and physician should strive to find a range of time when it would be most likely that a patient will die. In that range of time the close family may want to be summoned from out of town. In general, it can be said that the closer death is, the easier it is to predict the time course.

"If one declares medical futility,
one rules out the possibility of miracles."

This is a difficult issue. From a medical standpoint I would suggest that by removing medical support and allowing a natural progression toward life or death to occur, one can actually recognize a miracle if a reversal does occur. Otherwise, it is difficult to discern a miracle from a technological advance. It has been suggested that if one removes life-supporting medical interventions from a patient, then one might be "playing God." However, it would stand to reason that by keeping someone alive against natural forces at the end of his or her life, one would be much more likely to be playing God. By surrendering control over a patient's life support, one is releasing control to forces greater than oneself. By tightly controlling the bodily functions, one creates a very man-made, artificial situation.

"If the patient has been admitted to a particular hospital emergency room or office, their records are readily accessible and their case is well known to all the staff in attendance."

Unfortunately the medical system can be very chaotic. Charts are sometimes lost, and even if they are available the doctor or nurse may not be able to tell what truly occurred with previous visits. Therefore, it is important that the orchestration of end-of-life care be clearly documented. It is also important that the documents be carried by the patient's family as well as being stored in the medical setting.

"End-of-life care/active management of dying is essentially the same as euthanasia."

This is simply untrue. There are significant differences in styles of care. Please see Bert's discussion of this issue above to clarify the principles.

"A doctor would not do something to a patient unless it was in the person's best interest."

One must understand that the best interest of any one person is not easily definable. The phrase "best interest" is defined by one's value system. What may be in my best interest may not be in your best interest. The physician with pure motives may perform an act that is not in the best interest of a particular patient. This demonstrates the value of good communication and documentation. Each person has different wants, needs, and values. Without planning and knowledge, assumptions rather than truth may prevail.

"If my family member dies at home I will have bad memories to deal with."

This is an individual issue. Many people who have cared for their dying family members at home and watched them pass peacefully with good end-of-life care have expressed a tremendous sense of acceptance and resolution about the process and have actually been more able to get on with their lives. Some folks, however, are haunted by the memories and have trouble visiting the room where the loved one died. Therefore, it is very important to evaluate one's own feelings on the subject and anticipate how one will feel in the future. It would seem that by dealing with this issue ahead of time, and using good planning, whatever negative memories may occur will be lessened.

Notes

4

Create *an*
End-of-Life Care Plan

Lance writes . . .

By this point, you have developed skills to deal forthrightly with the concept of death and dying. You confronted denial and probably moved toward acceptance. You considered styles of decision-making. You thought about roles to be played by various individuals on behalf of the dying patient. You analyzed myths, and considered new ways of looking at a very serious issue. Just by virtue of the fact that you made it this far is a strong indicator that you have the courage and wisdom to do an admirable job as you work through the dying process, whether it is your own, or someone else's.

The next few steps are relatively easy by comparison. Our job at this point is to simply help you organize your thoughts into a meaningful end-of-life care plan. Obviously, every situation is different, so we must use generalities. Keep in mind what we have said many times before...the goal is to orchestrate a well-managed, peaceful, and comfortable death for the person for whom medical therapy is futile.

Rather than lengthy text, you may appreciate a clear, concise list of important considerations in your planning. In later chapters, you will find lengthy, descriptive advice on language and style that augments the following points:

- Call a family meeting. Include all appropriate people, especially the patient, if at all possible.

- Identify the surrogate, spokesperson, and leader. Often this will be the same person. If the patient is able and willing, he or she should be the leader and spokesperson.

- Clarify that medical futility has been reached and the patient or surrogate has decided to pursue comfort care as a priority.

- Relay known diagnostic and prognostic facts and opinions from the doctor, taking care to avoid speculation or elaboration.

- Give everyone a chance to voice their feelings regarding death and comfort care, in general and with regard to the dying person.

- Make sure the appropriate documents (for example, the living will, health care power of attorney, and Bedside Do Not Resuscitate order) have been filled out and signed. Place copies at the patient's bedside, at the doctor's office, and hospital and/or nursing home, as well as with the surrogate and other involved family members. It is wise to be over-prepared rather than under-prepared.

- Discuss with family and friends how much time and effort they are able to contribute to the care plan. Consider a schedule of attendants to be with the dying person. Consider bathing and hygiene: will the family handle it or will a professional, such as a nurse's aide, be hired? Identify needs and gaps to be discussed with the physician, social worker, and/or hospice people.

- Discuss funeral arrangements ahead of time to avoid confusion and angst during the turmoil and grief that may occur immediately after death.

- Make appointments with the doctor and hospice. Be prepared to make it clear that medical futility has been accepted, comfort measures are desired, and plans have been made to care for the patient as much as possible. Also be prepared to identify areas where help is needed. Do not be afraid to ask, as the professional may be aware of available resources that the layperson is not.

- By the time you have done these things, and taken some organized notes along the way, you will essentially have your plan in place. Review your notes and the situation, and write down an outline. We have provided a Notes Section at the end of this book to organize your information. This becomes the written representation of the end-of-life care plan. Everyone, from the patient to the physician, will be relieved to have addressed many of these issues ahead of time, and the patient will indeed receive much more focused and appropriate care than he or she would have otherwise.

- Once all that is in place, then turn your attention back to living. Within the time and energy remaining to the dying person, start imagining trips to be taken, visits to make, and conversations to be had. The team should focus on helping the person who is dying to move through the various stages of grieving and confession that Bert gave us, as well as helping the person to have fun and pleasure.

Notes

5

Implement *the* Care Plan You Created

Lance writes . . .

Imagine that you are planning a camping trip. If you do not plan well and subsequently fail to bring a tent, or sleeping bag, or matches, you may have a miserable time despite a beautiful setting. However, a well-planned trip, with appropriate gear, and everybody knowing their jobs, usually will result in a pleasurable experience, even if conditions are not perfect. The implementation of the plan becomes easy. One enjoys the time, rather than continually reacting to problems that arise because important planning steps were neglected. I personally would rather sit around a warm fire than spend hours scrambling to light it because no one remembered to pack matches.

Although dying is a much more serious issue than camping, the essential principle of good planning still holds true. By proactively anticipating pitfalls and making specific plans, many crises and pan-icky times are simply avoided and implementation of the end-of-life plan boils down to honest day-to-day living in the face of reality. The focus can be on pleasurable elements, such as remembering the person's life achievements and good relationships, physically holding and comforting the person and others, finding forgiveness and closure to loose ends, as well as enjoying play, humor, and storytelling. Consider implementation of the end-of-life plan to actually mean living as fully as one can for as long as one can.

The really good news is that by doing the previous work, you have essentially implemented the plan you created. Some maintenance and daily problem-solving will inevitably be required, but, as Bert noted, tackling small problems as they come up prevents the despair that occurs when one is confronted by a problem that became monstrous because it was ignored for too long.

Roles Assigned to Team Members

Maintenance of your plan will be facilitated by clarifying the roles assigned to various members of the team, as follows:

The individual who is dying. The individual becomes the focus. His or her job is simple: to let people help, and let them know what they need to do. If the dying person is able to communicate, he or she must find the courage to be honest so the rest of the team can know what to do next. If the person is incapacitated and unable to communicate, the surrogate, guardian, or caretaker of the moment must anticipate those needs.

The surrogate. The surrogate/spokesperson must be ready to stand firm to act on the patient's behalf even if there is dissent. The surrogate must have the courage to allow his charge to die when the time comes. In doing so, he will fulfill the plan and prevent the chaos that would expose the vulnerable dying person to unpleasant disruptions. He must assertively ask for pain medicine or additional comfort measures as the situation dictates.

Supporting friends and family. These people must be ready to be with the dying person, even during certain unpleasant times, and must keep promises regarding times when they will be with the person. There is a human tendency to get swept up in the planning and make statements about how much one can help out, and then later not be able to carry through to the level promised. It would be better to give a more conservative and realistic estimate of how much time and effort one can give. This will allow the planners to anticipate if additional services, such as home nursing or personal attendants, will be required.

The physician. The physician should guide the patient and family toward the most effective comfort care and services, such as hospice care. The physician should also continually provide a comforting but objective voice to keep the patient and family grounded in reality. He or she should invite office appointments to reaffirm the plan and the progress. In addition to ensuring quality care for the patient, the physician should keep an eye on the caregivers and point out signs of fatigue or depression, in order to protect the entire team and the effort. The physician must constantly address the patient's needs, and if the patient is incapacitated the physician should reinforce the surrogate as the representative voice of the patient.

Hospice/support services. The professional support should be accessible and down-to-earth with the patient and family. They should also look to the surrogate/spokesperson as the representative voice, and coordinate care with the physician. These people will provide frequent interaction and guidance to the patient and family. The patient/family should be prepared to call hospice first for issues such as increasing pain or deterioration in status.

Clergy/spiritual leader. This person will play a critical role and should be notified of the status of affairs throughout the process. Many families would opt to have the spiritual leader intricately involved throughout the planning while others would utilize them less formally. In any event, both scientific and anecdotal evidence is clear that attention to the patient's spiritual needs will decrease perceived pain and the need for narcotics, allowing the person to live more fully and contentedly during his or her remaining time.

Notes

6

Financial Planning

Lance writes . . .

I fell into a typical doctor trap as I was writing this book, and it ironically illustrates a point. Here I was trying to convey all this information I thought would be of practical benefit to the layperson. Like most doctors, I got caught up in medical knowledge and almost ignored the financial realities of health care. However, financial realities do profoundly influence the nature of health care in general and end-of-life care in particular. As we doctors do our work, we sometimes forget that our patients come from a variety of economic backgrounds, and the ability of patients to take our advice may be limited by financial constraints. The last thing dying persons or their families need is a monetary crisis. I have asked David Brookbank, President, Benchmark Life Strategies, LLC, to give you an overview of financial and insurance considerations for your planning.

Who Will Take Care of Us?

The information in this chapter is largely based on legislation and corporate policies and is therefore subject to frequent change.

David writes...

I learned many valuable lessons about life from my great-grandmother. She was born in 1897 and lived 104 years! I knew her for thirty-two of those years, and in addition to those lessons about life, she inadvertently taught me one of the most important lessons about dying.

When Granny became ill and unable to care for herself, the family was forced to make some very tough decisions. The first decision was to send her to the hospital, following a long bout with pneumonia. After the hospital stay, her physician recommended that she could be better cared for in a skilled facility. The family agreed, but the decision was not easy. With her extended family there were more than enough children and grandchildren to care for her at home. However, the question remained, would she receive the same care and treatment at home that she would receive in a skilled facility? Everyone agreed the facility was the best place for care, based on the circumstances and what was known to the family at the time.

Because Granny did not have private insurance she was at the mercy of the provider/payor of care (initially Medicare) to determine where she would receive this care. Fortunately for the family, or so we thought, a facility bed was available just a few blocks from the hospital. Within a few days the paperwork was completed and Granny was at her new home. Thankfully her children had the time and ability to sit with her frequently at the nursing facility to help with and observe her care. It was these observations that led to the family bringing her home to spend her last three years. The family also experienced the victory of a class action lawsuit that led to the facility being closed for their negligent treatment of patients.

I tell you this story not to scare you about skilled nursing facilities; there are many wonderful facilities available to us that provide excellent care. My point is that when Granny became ill, the choices of her care were very limited, and the family did not agree at all times on how her care was to be handled. Many of the decisions affecting her were made by people she didn't know. Given the opportunity, I'm sure she would have done things differently.

With the advancement of care facilities and private insurance, the choices of care when we become ill are far greater than they have been in the past. The one issue remaining for many of us when we become ill is that, at that point, we may be unable to determine the actual plan of care that we desire. This plan must be formulated, communicated, and in many cases funded, many years prior to our becoming ill.

Let's face it, every one of us will become ill at some point in our lives. Our final illness may only last a few seconds or many years. The point is that we do not have a crystal ball to determine how this will transpire. I'm sure this is why many of you are reading this book. With proper planning, the care we receive during our last days can be accomplished according to our desires and relieve some of the stressful decisions that would otherwise have to be made by our spouses and children.

Statistics show that most of us will live a long life. One of the consequences of this benefit is that at some point we are likely to need some type of long-term care. As defined by the National Association of Insurance Commissioners (NAIC), "long-term care" is [4]

> "The kind of help you need if you are unable to care for yourself because of a prolonged illness or disability. It can range from help with daily activities at home, such as bathing and dressing, to skilled nursing care in a nursing home. Long-term care is provided by home care agencies, senior centers, adult day care

---

[4] *Corporation for Long-Term Care Handbook.* Harley Gordon, 2003.

centers, traditional nursing homes, and *continuing care retirement communities. Family members can provide care as well."*

The need for care is normally based around the inability of the individual to perform at least two of the Activities of Daily Living, which include "bathing, eating, dressing, toileting, continence, and transferring," or "requiring substantial supervision to protect the individual from the threat to health and safety due to some cognitive impairment such as Alzheimer's or senile dementia."

It is no secret that the risk of a chronic illness increases with age. Care for this type of illness may last for many years before the patient actually passes away. In Granny's case, it lasted more than three years. It is not uncommon for the cost of care to exceed $100,000 per year, depending on the geographical area of the United States in which you live. Who provides us with this care? How do we pay for this care? (Note the word "we" because as I will illustrate later on in this chapter we are ultimately the ones paying for long-term care in one way or another.)

Here are some questions you can ask yourself: *What type of care will I need when I become ill? Who will provide the care I need when I become ill? Will it be skilled care? Or will it be non-skilled or custodial care* (care that is provided to those individuals needing help with performing the Activities of Daily Living or who need supervision due to a mental or cognitive impairment). And last but not least: *Who will pay for my care when I need it?*

These are not questions we spend a great deal of time pondering. For the most part we ask these questions after it is too late, and many of the options of care are no longer available. If we fail to plan out our desires for our personal care ahead of time we rely on others to make very important emotional and financial decisions for us. For many in this situation the decisions are made by emotionally and/or physically drained spouses or family members. The unhappy end result in many instances could have been avoided with a few hours of planning.

Today, we have numerous options for care. These include in-home care, assisted living facilities, adult day care, and skilled nursing facilities. I have listed these in order of preference by the majority of individuals with whom I consult.

Home Care

Given the option, most of us would prefer to be taken care of at home. Statistics tell us that approximately 80 percent of long-term care is administered in the home. The surroundings are familiar, and there is a certain peace about "home." Care in the home may be administered by professional home care nurses, nurse's aides, physicians, or family members. In-home care is not inexpensive. To afford the luxury of staying in your home when illness strikes will cost a pretty penny. As in the case with my great-grandmother, her care required that she have round-the-clock supervision (which was provided by her family), as well as a full-time nursing aide for eight hours a day. On some occasions her care also had to be administered by a physician and registered nurse. She had the luxury of having nine children to help with and administer her care, but most of us will not be that fortunate. The strain inflicted on a non-disabled spouse is enormous when that person is the primary caregiver. The responsibility of caring for a loved one in the final stages of life is more than a full-time job. It requires both physical and mental work on an ongoing basis. Without the assistance of social workers to design a plan of care, home health aides, homemaker aides, and nurse's aides, the task of care is virtually impossible.

Another critical element to allow the care recipient to remain at home is the use of adult day-care facilities. These services are usually community-based in nature and are normally open from eight to ten hours per day. The intent of the facility is to give the in-home caregiver (normally the spouse or adult children) respite care. In other words, a daily break from the routines of caring for the recipient. Adult day care is usually administered for those individuals who need help with some form of the Activities of Daily Living other than toileting. The cost for this type of care can be quite expensive. Depending on the geographical location, cost of care can exceed $100 a day in many areas of the country.

Assisted Living

Assisted living facilities are available to provide care for those individuals who still may be able to get through the normal routines of the day but require some assistance with the Activities of Daily Living. The environment is typically that of being "at home" with apartment-style living. The cost for assisted-living facilities (again depending on geography) starts around $2,000 a month and increases from there. The average stay in this type of facility is currently thirty months.

When the term "long-term care" is mentioned, people most often associate this with care provided strictly at a nursing home or a skilled nursing facility. In the past that may have been true; however, these facilities are providing care in a much different role today. With the development of modern medicine, the ability to stay in the home and receive care for an extended period of time, and the development of adult day-care and assisted-living facilities, the identity of skilled nursing facilities has dramatically changed. The new role for these facilities is to provide for the "sickest of the sick, or those who have no support services or family in the community," according to Harley Gordon, President of CLTC Corporation. The skilled nursing facility's role is to provide the level of care that is designed to rehabilitate the patient in order to return home. For this reason, it should be no surprise that in many cases involving elderly persons, the next step to rehabilitation from a hospital stay is to a skilled nursing facility. However, we know from experience that this rehabilitation does not always occur, and the patient becomes a permanent resident of the facility.

Hospice

Hospice is a very unique service that provides care for those individuals on a terminally ill prognosis. The organization focuses on the care itself rather than the cure for the illness. Their services include providing emotional support for the family members of the patient. Personally, I have heard nothing but positive things about hospice care and those who work for these organizations. It takes a very special person to help care for a terminally ill patient, especially in the final stages of the illness. Hospice workers generally bring about a very noticeable level of comfort for both the patient and the family members. Hospice provides services in either a facility setting or in-home care.

Most insurance policies including Medicare and Medicaid have a hospice benefit. All that is usually required to activate this benefit is a doctor's prognosis that the life expectancy is 6 months or less. Please check with your insurance company or agent for specific details.

Retirement Communities

Community care retirement communities are another option for many elderly individuals and couples long before care is ever needed. These communities are usually run by non-profit organizations or religious institutions. The care in this type of setting ranges from totally independent living to assisted-living care to on-site skilled nursing facilities. These communities offer excellent lifestyle changes for a single elderly person or an elderly couple who have concerns about their future care. Residents can lead a very active lifestyle with the peace of mind that care will be available when needed. The entry fees into this type of facility are substantial. (I am not aware of any facility currently charging less than six figures to enter.) A monthly maintenance charge is assessed as well. In many cases, depending on the level of care needed throughout your stay, this monthly charge may be increased. I normally caution clients who are looking at these types of communities to be aware of the community's ability to raise monthly fees, as well as to explore the non-refundable entry fees associated with many communities.

One of my good friends lives in one of these communities. He was recently sharing with me that due to the portfolio performance (or lack thereof) of the non-profit that owns the facility, the monthly maintenance fees had jumped from $1,100 per month to over $2,000 per month for residents. Many of the residents feel they are stuck in this particular situation because they are at the mercy of the governing non-profit. The last time we spoke, my friend notified me that the residents had filed a lawsuit to fight the current and any future increases. My question is what happens when a facility of this type becomes insolvent? Where do the residents go? What recourse do they have? For these reasons I must urge anyone considering a retirement community of this type to use extreme caution before making this decision.

Medicare

At this point I will again pose the question: *Who will pay for my care when I need it?* As I mentioned before, *we* are ultimately the ones paying for our own care. In the United States we have a wonderful system called Medicare. I am sure that most of you reading this book have heard about this program. Many of you are probably Medicare recipients.

In the right setting, the Medicare system with the proper accompanying supplement will pay for the health care needs for most senior citizens and qualified disabled participants with two exceptions: prescription drugs and long-term care.

With most Medicare supplement policies there are no benefits for prescription drugs unless the recipient has plan G, plan I or plan J. Neither of these two plans will provide for more than 50 percent of extended outpatient prescription drugs. The maximum annual benefit of $3,000 is found under plan J. Should you be covered under a Medicare HMO plan you probably have little or no prescription drug coverage. It is extremely important to discuss the costs of these drugs due to their impact on a long-term care illness.

The second limitation that Medicare has involves long-term care services. If I had a dollar for every time a client said to me in the initial meeting: "If I get sick and need care my Medicare will take care of my needs," I would be able to...well, I would be able to do many things. The point is that most of us believe Medicare will pay the bills when we become ill and need care, but guess what? The time when most people find out that Medicare *will not pay* for the care they need is when it is too late and they need care!

Medicare divides care into skilled and non-skilled (custodial) care. Medicare only covers services defined as skilled with a few catches. Medicare Part A will cover care that is provided in the skilled nursing facility arena. Medicare will pay the full cost of care for the first twenty days *if:*

1. The patient has received inpatient hospital care for at least three consecutive nights and entered the skilled facility within thirty days of that hospital stay.

2. The patient must be entering the skilled facility for the same medical reason for which he or she was hospitalized.

I should also mention at this point that the patient must show some potential for improvement of health, or Medicare will not pay for care.

After twenty days in the skilled facility, Medicare charges a daily deductible of $109.50 a day (in 2004), from day 21 through day 100. Medicare recipients with Medicare supplement plans C through J will receive the benefit of their supplement paying the $109.50 a day through day 100. After the 100 days, Medicare pays nothing for skilled nursing facility coverage. The patient could receive another 100 days of benefits if he or she does not require hospital care or skilled nursing care for sixty days. The new benefit period is rarely utilized as Medicare applies to skilled nursing care.

Prior to July 1, 1998, Medicare paid for skilled facility coverage on a fee-for-service basis. The average skilled facility stay paid by Medicare was fifty days. Medicare thought that appropriate accounting was not being done and the system was being abused. Therefore, on July 1, 1998, Medicare implemented a flat-fee payment system. The result was an automatic reduction in the number of days funded by Medicare in a skilled facility—it was cut by more than half. In other words, overnight the skilled nursing facility industry went from being a cash cow to being insolvent. Almost every major skilled nursing home chain has become bankrupt due to the fee adjustment by Medicare.

It should also be noted that prior to January 1998 both Medicare Part A and Medicare Part B covered an unlimited number of home health care visits. As you can imagine, many of our elected officials believed that the system was being abused by for-profit Medicare-certified home health agencies. They were right! The Medicare system changed on January 1, 1998 with the Balanced Budget Act of 1997. Currently Medicare will reimburse for home care under the following conditions: [5]

1. The beneficiary must be confined to the home.

2. The beneficiary must require skilled nursing care or physical or speech therapy on an intermittent basis; or, if they had earlier met these criteria and received home care but no longer meet them, they must continue to need occupational therapy.

3. A plan for furnishing the home care services must be established and periodically reviewed by a physician.

4. The beneficiary must be under a physician's care when receiving these services.

Once the above criteria are met, Medicare Part A will cover home health care to the extent of medically necessary skilled care, home health aide services, and medical supplies. The benefit period is for as long as the beneficiary meets the Medicare criteria for home health care benefits. Services are covered at 100 percent of the Medicare approved amount and 80 percent of the Medicare approved amount for durable

---

[5] 42 U.S.C.S. 1395(a) (2) (C)

medical equipment. Medicare Part B covers the services not covered in Part A, which includes part-time skilled care, home health aide services, durable medical equipment, and other medical supplies and services. The beneficiary is eligible to receive benefits subject to the Balanced Budget Act of 1997. The problem with planning for Medicare to pay for your care is the fact that it is very tough to qualify and maintain the qualifications necessary to receive benefits. You have given up control and the future of your care lies within the hands of our elected officials!

I also recommend that most individuals steer clear of Medicare HMO plans due to the financial strains facing these organizations. Medicare HMOs take the financial risk from the federal government and shoulder the burden of expense themselves. Fewer and fewer physicians are accepting HMO payments and many physicians are now suing HMO plans due to delayed claim payments, arbitrarily changing fee structures, and denying necessary medical care for patients. The result is that many traditional insurers are shying away from the financial responsibility of funding the care. Switching from an HMO to a traditional Medicare supplement should be handled cautiously. I highly recommend a consultation with an insurance agent or broker before making the decision to switch.

Who pays for Medicare? You and I do through our taxes. *What does Medicare pay for with regard to long-term care?* Nothing unless you qualify. Should you qualify, benefits are limited and your future is determined by legislation.

Medicaid

What about Medicaid? You may have heard that Medicaid will pay for everything associated with your long-term care needs. You are right! It will pay for most everything; however, you must first qualify. I'm sure for some of you I am preaching to the choir. You may have a loved one who has had the unfortunate experience of spending his or her assets down to the poverty level in order to qualify for this wonderful service. *What? Are you telling me that I must liquidate everything in order to receive this benefit?* Well, pretty much. In order to qualify for Medicaid services you must understand your particular state's rules regarding qualification. In general, Medicaid divides your assets into three categories:

1. **Countable assets.** These are assets that are controlled by the applicant for Medicaid. These assets must be liquidated or spent to pay for the cost of the applicant's care. These include:

   - All forms of cash
   - Bonds
   - Stocks
   - IRA, Keogh, 401-k, 403-b, and 529 plans
   - All general investments
   - All tax-qualified pension plans (if applicant is retired)
   - Deferred annuities (if not annuitized)
   - All life insurance with cash surrender value (if death benefit exceeds $1,500)
   - Vacation homes/property
   - Investment property

2. **Non-countable assets.** As the name indicates, these assets are not used in determining eligibility. These include:

   - A small amount of cash ($3,000 or less—varies by state)
   - A primary residence—only if the spouse lives in the home, the applicant intends to return home, or a dependent child under the age of twenty-one, blind or disabled lives in the home
   - Pre-paid funeral services
   - Term life insurance
   - Certain business assets
   - Car for personal use
   - Personal items

3. Inaccessible assets—assets that have been transferred by either placing them in a trust or giving them away.

Medicaid will allow the spouse who does not require long-term care to keep a minimum amount of assets and income. Some couples believe that various assets will not become "countable assets" if certain conditions exist. For example, many couples believe that a premarital agreement will protect assets from being a countable asset. Premarital arrangements will not protect assets from being countable assets.

When planning for many seniors I am quick to learn that many people are ready and willing to give away assets to qualify for Medicaid. The problem here is that the state government realizes this as well. Advisors beware! I believe that Senator Kennedy and Senator Kassenbaum addressed the transfer of assets in a very clear manner in 1996. The Health Insurance Portability and Accountability Act of 1996 says: [6]

> *"Whoever...for a fee knowingly and willfully counsels or assists an individual to dispose of assets (including by any transfer in trust) in order for the individual to become eligible for medical assistance under a State plan under title XIX, if disposing of the assets results in the imposition of a period of ineligibility for such assistance under section 1917(c)...shall...be guilty of a misdemeanor and upon conviction be fined not more than $10,000 or imprisoned for not more than one year or both."*

As an advisor, two things in that paragraph leap off the page—the words "ten thousand dollars" and "imprisoned." For the record, let me state that I have not, nor will I ever assist a client, family member, or even an enemy in moving assets in order to qualify for Medicaid. Beware of the planner who advises you that placing assets into a living trust or a revocable trust will help you qualify for Medicaid! They are dead wrong—the main function of a living trust is to protect assets

---

[6] 42 U.S.C.S.1320a-7b (a)

from probate and keeps matters private. It does nothing to protect the assets from being "counted" toward the Medicaid spend-down!

Most people have the misconception that Medicaid is this system that actually takes your money and uses it to pay for your care. Actually the Medicaid system has the right to place a lien on certain assets to recover expenses; however, the actual "paying" of funds takes place in what is called an ineligibility period where one must "spend down" assets to qualify for state benefits. Assets transferred to an individual will carry a three-year look-back provision, while assets transferred to an irrevocable trust will carry a five-year look-back provision. Medicaid has a very nice formula for calculating the ineligibility period for an individual. During the ineligibility period, the individual must pay for the cost of care out of pocket. As you can imagine, if an individual has transferred assets out of his or her name, paying for the cost of care might not be easy.

In summary, Medicaid is a fine program set in place to take care of the indigent. If you have any significant assets I recommend not trying to qualify for Medicaid. There are other alternatives. For a listing of helpful information with regard to your state's Health Insurance Assistance Programs as well as your state's Department of Insurance contact numbers, please visit our website at www.benchmarklifestrategies.com.

Veteran's Admin (VA)

Many veterans believe the Veterans Administration will pay for their care. In most cases the VA classifies all veterans into "priority groups." Each group is rated based on service-related disabilities, and care is provided based on where the individual fits within the group. The bottom line is that the VA does not offer long-term care to most of our veterans.

Long-Term Care Insurance

Self-funding is a viable option for the wealthy; however, why would someone want to pay for expenses out of pocket at 100 percent when they could purchase a long-term care (LTC) insurance policy for pennies on the dollar *and* potentially tax-deduct part or all of the premium. The long-term care policies of today are molded from ideas by the National Association of Insurance Commissioners (NAIC). Policies are regulated by each state's Department of Insurance. Each policy *must* meet certain specifications and criteria in order to be sold in the marketplace. In the early days of LTC insurance there was abuse of the elderly population by a money-hungry sales force and severe limits on contract language. Policies did not typically cover Alzheimer's disease. Many policies (like Medicare) also required hospitalization before benefits would be paid. Policy language was very murky and distorted. To remedy this problem, in 1993 the NAIC came up with standard policy provisions that are on all LTC policies sold today. As an example, there is now no prior hospitalization requirement before benefits begin, and Alzheimer's disease as well as severe cognitive impairments are covered under all policies. Other provisions that make coverage more attractive to purchase are:

- Thirty-day free look at all LTC policies

- A time limit of two years for pre-existing conditions

- Policies are guaranteed renewable, which means that the carrier must renew the policy regardless of claims experience

- Policy owners are given the opportunity to protect the policy benefits against rising care costs with an inflation protection rider

- Policies cover home health care as well as community-based care

Typically, there are two triggers to qualify for benefits under a tax-qualified long-term care policy. The first deals with the physical inability to perform two of the Activities of Daily Living (again, these consist of bathing, eating, dressing, toileting, continence, and transferring). Each insurance contract will differ slightly as to its definition of "assistance" with these activities. The second trigger deals with a cognitive impairment such as Alzheimer's or dementia. The NAIC model drastically improved long-term care coverage and made it much more consumer friendly.

After one of the benefit triggers have been satisfied, the individual must meet the policy's elimination period or waiting period before payment of benefits begin. Simply put, the elimination period is the number of days an individual must wait before receiving benefits form his or her policy. Elimination/waiting periods vary from "0 days" to "two years." Obviously, the shorter elimination period will result in a higher premium. Each case and individual needs are different. Many people choose to take the risk and "self fund" the elimination period or they take the risk of Medicare paying for the first 100 days of care. Please keep in mind that it is very difficult to qualify for the 100-day benefit from Medicare. After benefits begin, premiums are usually waived for the time period that the insured is on claim.

A good long-term care policy should contain the following provisions in addition to paying for skilled nursing facility care:

1. Home care (sometimes referred to as in-home care). This provision should cover services necessary for care that are provided in the home environment. Many people associate home care with care that is provided on a 24-hour basis. Coverage provided on an around-the-clock basis is much more expensive than skilled nursing facility coverage. Home care provides the professional services and respite care in order to give the primary caregiver a much deserved break.

2. Benefits for care in an assisted living facility when applicable.

3. Adult day care. For those primary caregivers who typically work outside the home, this type of care is an answered prayer. Many

individuals who need daily supervision but are still able to interact with others will find this type of care very helpful. These care centers are usually open Monday through Friday.

4. Inflation protection for the rising costs of care. Usually policies will either have a 5 percent compound or 5 percent simple inflation factor, which will rise each year to keep pace with the rising costs of care. I normally recommend the compound inflation factor for individuals who are under the age of seventy. From the ages of seventy-one through seventy-six, simple inflation protection is recommended; however, there is no one set model for policy design. For clients who are seventy-seven and older, I generally recommend a higher daily benefit due to the dramatic cost of inflation protection at those ages. Each individual is different, with different needs and desires. The agent as well as the client must perform due diligence through the buying process to be sure the policy coverage is suitable for the individual.

Long-term care policies will either fall under the categories of reimbursement, indemnity, or cash benefit. A reimbursement contract will do exactly as it states. Let's look at an example.

Say you have an LTC policy that provides a daily reimbursement benefit of $150. You begin receiving benefits, and you incur actual expenses of $100 in a given day. Your contract will pay $100, in other words reimbursing you for the actual expenses incurred. The reimbursement contract is the most economical of the three types of contracts.

An indemnity policy will pay for the entire monthly or daily amount of service provided while on claim. As an example:

Say you have a LTC policy that provides a daily indemnity benefit of $150. You begin receiving benefits, and you incur actual expenses of $100 in a given day. Your contract will pay $150 regardless of the fact that the cost of care for that day was only $100.

The extra $50 could be used to offset the expenses of any incidentals such as medications, bed linens, and so forth.

A cash benefit policy does not require that any service be given in any one particular day in order to receive benefits. Once the benefit triggers have been enacted, the policyholder will receive the entire monthly or daily benefit agreed upon in the contract. For example:

Say you have an LTC policy that provides a daily cash benefit of $150. You begin receiving benefits due to satisfying a benefit policy trigger. You will receive $150 each day you are on claim regardless if care was administered.

Obviously this type of contract is the most expensive of the three due to the liberal benefit.

As you can expect, literally hundreds of insurance companies rushed into the market with their sites set on the 77 million baby boomers as their targets. Since that time many insurers have decided to exit the marketplace and to sell their existing policies to larger companies willing to take the risk. Many policyholders have found themselves experiencing increases in premiums from carriers in order for the particular company to meet reserve and claim obligations. Due to the constantly changing environment, I have compiled a checklist to review when considering a long-term care policy:

1. Did I contact the agent representing this policy or did the agent contact me? Countless numbers of solicitations are being made each day. Make sure you trust the person with whom you are working. Referrals are a great way to find an agent.

2. Is the agent representing only one company rather than showing me a variety of carriers to allow me to decide which one best fits my needs? If the agent represents only one company they probably do not have your best interest in mind.

3. Do I need as much coverage as is being presented? Many agents will not look at the client's entire picture before making a recommendation. They fail to include factors such as current assets and income used to help offset the cost of care. I can't tell you the number of times I have met with a client who has been shown $150/day of benefit when in reality they need much less.

4. What are the financial ratings of the insurance company? Financial insolvency is a hazard and a risk of choosing a company with a low rating. Check several rating sources. These include Moody's, Standard & Poor's, and A. M. Best. I recommend an "A" rating or higher.

5. Can I afford the coverage? Again, do not be oversold!

6. Does the policy provide for home care? If so what is the monthly or daily amount designated for care? Many agents will reduce the amount of home care to one-half of the cost for skilled nursing care. Beware of this act! I normally recommend that home care benefits be at the same level as skilled care benefits. In addition, I like to see a "0 day" waiting period on home care. The odds on your needing care in the home are much greater initially than skilled care.

7. What is my waiting or elimination period? How long will you have to wait before benefits begin? One common misconception by agents is that Medicare will cover the first 100 days in a facility—*this is wrong, and you will most likely lose this bet!* You should consider how long you could afford to pay out-of-pocket for your care, and then choose the appropriate elimination period, while keeping in mind the appropriate cost you are willing to pay for the coverage.

8. Does the policy have an inflation rider to protect against the increasingly high costs associated with care? Do I need inflation protection?

9. Has the carrier ever increased premiums on current policyholders? If so, how many times and how much were the increases? This will give you a good gauge as to how the company is doing financially with regard to pricing and future increases that you may receive as a policyholder.

10. If I am turned down for coverage with one carrier does this mean that I can't get coverage? Not necessarily. Carriers vary on underwriting decisions. However, if you are receiving care for an illness you can bet that you will not be allowed to purchase new or additional coverage. Important note: If you can qualify for coverage, can afford the coverage, and know that you need the coverage—it is best that you act while you are healthy. I have often received calls from people wanting to purchase coverage, and it is already too late. Their health has deteriorated to the point that no insurer would touch them.

I have tried to inform you, the reader, with enough knowledge to make an educated decision regarding the care of you and your family. The industry surrounding care for the elderly changes daily. It would be impossible to cover all of the bases in a mere chapter of this book, but I hope I have brought a new insight to each of you as it pertains to long-term care and how *we* pay for it because, as I have proven in this chapter, *we* are the ones who will pay!

———

More information is available at: **www.benchmarklifestrategies.com** or call us at 1-866-828-5104 or 1-336-856-7900. You may also e-mail me at **david b@benchmarklifestrategies.com.**

———

We encourage you to use the extensive note section
at the back of the book

7

Narrative Case Examples

(All names in Cases 1-4 are changed to protect confidentiality.)

Lance writes . . .

—— CASE 1: MR. MILLER ——

I met Fred Miller and his wife, Jane, in the emergency department during my residency. It was a night when I was on call for the Family Medicine service. This was relatively early in my medical career, and his case taught me a tremendous amount.

The couple had been married for over thirty years and had enjoyed good health and vitality for most of that time. Jane was sixty-seven and still healthy and mentally sharp. Fred was sixty-nine and had been bed-bound for three years due to a massive stroke. In the emergency department, Jane told me tearfully about the stroke and the subsequent three years. Fred had gone from an active traveler to a completely dependent person in a matter of hours. He had lost all ability to speak or follow instructions and responded only to very deep stimuli, with small movements of his right arm. Despite Jane's excellent care and constant attention, about a year after the stroke Fred began to suffer the inevitable problems of the bed-bound patient. He had developed several pneumonias and urinary tract infections, which had become increasingly difficult to treat. The skin over his buttocks and heels began to break down and developed sores that did not heal. Although he could not feed himself, or even indicate hunger or thirst, Jane was able to spoon-feed Fred without undue trouble.

Then, two years after the stroke, Fred stopped accepting nutrition by mouth. He simply stopped chewing and swallowing. At that point, Jane knew that Fred's condition was deteriorating. In fact, she had an awareness and acceptance that Fred was ready to die. Not knowing what to do, Jane asked Fred's physician for advice. She told me the response was worded, "If we don't put a feeding tube in place, he will die.'" This was a critical and unfortunate moment for Fred and Jane. Jane knew Fred had never wanted to be kept alive by artificial means if he ever became unable to live independently or to interact with his environment. However, when faced with the choice of either using a feeding tube or "letting Fred die," Jane could not bear the guilt of choosing the latter. So, a feeding tube was placed through Fred's abdominal wall into his stomach, and Jane learned how to give liquid nutrition using the tube.

Over the next year, Fred's visits to the emergency room and hospitalizations increased due to recurrent infections and complications related to the feeding tube. Jane related that the doctors usually guided her in solving the immediate problem, but no one helped her in planning for Fred's inevitable death. The big picture was avoided. She felt too guilty to ask about withdrawing support or not treating the infections, in order to allow Fred to die naturally. She became depressed and felt isolated, and her self-care suffered.

It was about one year after initial placement of the tube that I met Fred and Jane in the emergency department. Jane had called EMS in desperation after Fred had unconsciously pulled the feeding tube from his stomach and had taken in no fluid or nutrition for over a day. Fred was gaunt, dehydrated, contracted, wearing a diaper, and basically unresponsive to anything except deeply painful stimuli. The emergency physician had begun giving intravenous (IV) fluids. Basic lab work revealed a severe urinary tract infection. IV antibiotics had also been started to treat the infection. No one had actually spoken with Jane about a complete plan of care prior to the testing or treatment. Jane later told me that she knew Fred was ready to die and wished treatment had not been started, but was afraid to say so. After reviewing Fred's chart and performing a physical exam, it was clear to me that the man was a "victim of the system." In other words, he needed comfort care during his impending natural death, but instead he had received inappropriate life-sustaining measures.

At that stage in my training I recognized that Fred's life was over and that further medical intervention was not only futile, but would prolong and increase his suffering. I knew that well-orchestrated comfort measures and withdrawal of further treatment or artificial feedings was the appropriate path. I could also sense that Jane felt the same way. However, my knowledge and confidence were not yet working in unison, and I admitted Fred to the floor, promising Jane I would continue antibiotics and "do all I could" for Fred. Even then I had a sense that Jane felt as I did, that Fred was ready to pass, but I did not yet know how to get to the heart of the matter.

On the ward, Fred's infection did improve somewhat with the antibiotics and hydration, and we began to make plans to have his feeding tube replaced. Of course, his mental and physical state showed no overall improvement. My instincts and training told me it was wrong to replace the tube, but I was unsure of the right way to address the issue with Jane. Would she accuse me of being unfeeling? Of wanting her to be alone? Of trying to euthanize her husband? What if I was wrong? Who was I to decide? What right did I have to play God?

Finally, I decided I was two things...this man's doctor and a human being with a sense of reality. I approached Jane at the bedside and said, "May I speak to you outside?"

We found a quiet room to sit and talk. I told Jane we had plans to replace the feeding tube the next day, and then Fred could go home on antibiotics. She gave a neutral nod of understanding. I paused and said, "I don't want to offend you by what I am about to say...but, I am not sure that putting the tube back in is the right thing to do." Jane looked me in the eye and indicated I could continue. "He has been in this state a long time, and he is getting worse, not better." She nodded, and I said, "Do you think continuing to keep him alive this way is what he would have wanted?"

The anguish, the guilt, and the exhaustion were evident on her face. She paused, and then asked, "What else can we do?"

Her return question let me know she was open to other options, and that she was ready to hear of them. Knowledge then gave me confidence. We talked at length about arranging comfort measures and withdrawing medical support, allowing Fred to die peacefully. To my surprise, Jane broke down into tears of relief, as well as sadness, and thanked me repeatedly for bringing up a subject that had never been discussed. She expressed her profound frustration that had built up over the past three years, and the guilt that came from watching Fred suffer and being part of the process that kept him alive in such a state. She sensed my own reaction to all this. In a grandmotherly way, she hugged me and said, "You did the right thing, you gave me choices...I did not know what could happen." In that moment it was clear that my own fears had been as unfounded as hers. We both learned something that day.

We stopped the IV fluids and antibiotics. We cancelled the gastro-enterologist (digestive tract specialist) consultation for the feeding tube placement. Jane made preparations to have Fred back at home with hospice care. I wrote orders to make sure Fred had adequate morphine and sedatives to keep him comfortable. I found myself hovering at his bedside with Jane. As discharge planning proceeded, Fred quickly declined. His infection returned, and his blood pressure dropped as he dehydrated again. Jane asked me if he could stay in the hospital to die because she feared the transfer to home would disturb him. She regretted he was not already at home, but she felt the ambulance ride would be worse. I knew it would not be long and agreed with her.

I was at the bedside with her when he took his last breath. He was comfortable and quiet. His lips were moist because of excellent nursing care. He simply came to a stop. That is how I describe it. He took one last, slow breath and then lost his color. My attending physician, also present, gave me a nod and left me with the couple. Jane looked at me. I listened for a heartbeat, felt for a pulse, and looked for pupil response. Sensing none, I simply said, "He is gone." She gave my hand a squeeze, and I left them together.

When Jane emerged from the room she looked calm and peaceful, less sad than I had seen her. She accepted a small prescription of mild sleeping pills from me in case she had trouble at night, but said she probably would not need them. I felt the same peace. It was a feeling of quiet victory and of harmony. We both knew we had formed a team to meet a difficult task. We had succeeded.

—— CASE 2: MR. SMITH ——

Later on in my medical training I was confronted with a memorable case. It was a very difficult time, and I think the patient suffered much more because of some decisions that were made along the way. This case occurred in the latter half of my residency. I had developed some sense of organization about the dying process, and I was becoming confident in my ability to assist families during this time. This patient, we will call him John Smith, had suffered a stroke about four years prior to my meeting him. Before that he had already been showing signs of dementia, probably related to a long history of alcohol abuse.

By the family's description, even before the stroke he had been losing some ability to take care of himself due to some forgetfulness and lapses in his thought processes. After the stroke his dementia became much worse and he lost most of his motor skills. For the last four years he had been cared for at home but was essentially bed-bound. The family was very protective of him and brought him to the emergency room whenever he got sick. They had not been able to consolidate his care to one single doctor. For several years, as he developed urinary tract infections or pneumonias, he would get immediate treatment at the emergency room. He would then be taken home and would be relatively stable for a few months until the same problems arose again. Because he was bed-bound he began to develop pressure sores on his buttocks, elbows, and heels. Over the last two years the sores had become worse. He was actually hospitalized several times to treat the infections associated with the sores and had to have surgical debridement (cleaning) of the wounds.

I was asked to admit this patient from the emergency room to the hospital due to more complications of the problems listed above. I had never seen the patient before, and he came to me through our "unassigned call" list. (Each hospital emergency department has a list of local physicians who take turns admitting patients who do not have established physicians.) By the time I admitted him he had an obvious pneumonia in his right lower lung, which was making his breathing difficult, and two of his bedsores were over ten centimeters in diameter. One had deteriorated all the way down to his lower sacral (buttocks) bone. The sores were exquisitely painful as the raw tissue and bone were exposed; however, this time they were not truly infected. Mr. Smith had no control over his bowels or bladder and so wore an adult diaper.

After taking history from the family and performing an exam, it was clear that the wounds were never going to get better. It was also apparent that he was in tremendous pain. He had no ability to communicate except to moan, almost scream, loudly when the wounds were touched. Because of his own waste products and the chronic wounds, and despite the family's attempt to keep him clean, he had an odor about him that can only be described as decay. His muscles were contracted, and he was emaciated. His teeth were in a state of painful decay. There were obvious cavities and several loose teeth. Due to the pneumonia, his breathing was shallow and the lungs sounded "wet" on the right side. His oxygen saturation was low. As I read his chart, I found this was the fourth pneumonia he'd had in the same lung. It is well known in medicine that when a human being is unable to move himself around, change position, or expand the lungs, then pneumonia is an inevitable outcome. Even when treated with antibiotics, such pneumonias will occur over and over again.

Before going back to speak to the family, I felt a sense of apprehension because it was clear they were not working in unison. Some members obviously had the mindset that the doctors should do "everything" to save this patient's life. Other family members did not seem to agree but did not look as if they wanted to speak up. Before leaving the bedside to approach the family, it was clear to me that treating this pneumonia would be a futile intervention. It would do nothing except extend this man's life a few more months and prolong his obvious pain and suffering.

We sat and talked. I tried to help them understand the futility of his condition, but their reaction was opposite to what I had come to expect. Even though they acknowledged Mr. Smith was in pain and not really getting better, they insisted the pneumonia be treated and the wounds be cleaned again. It seemed that guilt and some sense of obligation were the primary motivating factors behind their position. They were not able to release the guilt or overcome the other barriers, and I was not yet confident enough to take myself off the case. I admitted the patient that night and began antibiotics. In the morning, we requested a surgical consultation to debride (surgically clean) the wounds. We also asked the Wound Care team to help with the long-term problems. The family seemed temporarily satisfied, and our team resolved to speak with them again regarding the long-term care for this patient.

Over the next few days Mr. Smith slowly recovered from his pneumonia. High doses of powerful antibiotics were required to treat what would be a simple pneumonia in a healthier individual. Cultures revealed the presence of strains of bacteria that were resistant to most antibiotics. This in itself caused alarm because the repeated antibiotics had essentially bred these dangerous, resistant bacteria. Now they were being spread around the hospital only to colonize and possibly infect others. Mr. Smith, despite large doses of morphine and other pain medications, never seemed comfortable. He moaned continuously. The surgeons did the best they could with the wounds, but their options were limited. The wounds would not be able to heal because he would always be putting pressure on them in bed. The Wound Care team provided various dressings and topical ointments for superficial care. Everyone realized we were only slowing the inevitable.

I was surprised to find the family was not gaining acceptance of the futility of this patient's case. When I brought up the subject of withdrawing support again they became angry. One accused me of being a "quack." The situation was getting out of control, and I was torn between the care plan I knew was in the best interest of the patient and the wishes of the family. Many months later, when I had a chance to reflect on this case, I vowed that henceforth I would act in the best interest of the patient, even if the family did not agree initially. If they could not accept my clinical decisions, I would be ready to take myself off the case and find a new physician for the patient. Fortunately, this has never been necessary because families usually recognize when a doctor is standing up for the right plan of care. At the time, our next step was to ask for some second opinions from other physicians and the hospital's ethics committee. The consensus was that medical care was futile.

Again, to my surprise and remorse, this was not enough to convince the family. Despite our better judgment, we continued treatments for the pneumonia and the wounds. After ten days, the patient was stable enough to go home. The family expressed reluctant thanks and refused a hospice consultation. Two weeks later, Mr. Smith was back in the emergency room and I was called down to see him again. He had a temperature of 105°F and his breathing was labored, shallow, and deteriorating. His eyes were wide open with fear, and his lungs were saturated with pus and fluid. His wounds looked even worse, and it was obvious he was in shock from the overwhelming infection. The family was once again present and insisted that we put a breathing tube and other resuscitative measures into place. As we tried to begin this process, Mr. Smith's vital signs deteriorated rapidly. He died before we could perform any resuscitative interventions.

When I delivered the news, some of the more quiet family members showed relief on their faces. Those who had insisted on "everything" being done actually appeared angry with me that Mr. Smith had died. This case was one of the most unsettling and difficult I have ever known. I would consider it an example of where everyone loses. Most importantly, Mr. Smith suffered and was in pain for a long time. The family members who apparently had wanted to let him die, but did not speak up, had to deal with the guilt of knowing their family member had suffered needlessly while they said nothing. The family members who had refused to accept the reality and the futility carried away a sense of misdirected anger that would hinder their grief and healing.

I, of course, felt terrible about the whole thing and carried away a sense of guilt and anger as well. I must have reflected on this case hundreds of times and never felt much better about it. However, if this case serves to prevent others from suffering needlessly, it will have meaning.

Although this case was disturbing, it was among my best learning experiences. It humbled me and made me reevaluate my actions. It should be emphasized that I am not angry with the family. They were experiencing frightening and confusing emotions. This case reinforced the need in our society for guidance and awareness regarding end-of-life care. I felt that if this family had had a chance to read and gain some understanding prior to the crisis, they would have been able to accept reality and work productively to improve it.

—— CASE 3: REV. FISK ——

I found the next case to be among the most interesting and rewarding thus far in my medical career. I was admitting patients from the emergency department to our Family Medicine service. The ED called me down to evaluate an elderly gentleman who had suffered a ruptured cerebral aneurysm (a blood vessel had ruptured in his brain) a year before. This had left him in a completely vegetative state with global paralysis and no meaningful interactions. Since then he had experienced a number of urinary tract infections and pneumonias. He had been cared for immaculately at his home by his family. It turned out he was formerly a Southern Baptist preacher, and he had enjoyed significant standing in the community for many years. He had a large family who loved him dearly.

This particular night he had been vomiting and had a fever due to a severe urinary tract infection. Being farther along in my training, I was comfortable immediately addressing the "big picture" with the family. They were receptive to a discussion about a change in the focus of his care, but because not all the family was present, they were unable to reach a decision. We decided to admit Rev. Fisk. The plan was clear. We would offer some fluids and antibiotics immediately to keep him alive until we could assemble the family and have a more complete discussion about end-of-life plans. The family was not in denial, they simply had not been able to come to a consensus, actually due to the fact that they were so respectful of each other's opinions that no one wanted to speak for the missing family members.

The next day we had a family meeting. There were twelve siblings present. The patient's wife had died the year before. Since the siblings were the primary caretakers, they had a rotation schedule established, taking turns living in Rev. Fisk's house, instead of their own, in order to take care of him.

When we sat down to talk, the medical team noted the increasing frequency and severity of Rev. Fisk's infections and the failure of more and more antibiotics to treat them. That led into a fairly advanced conversation about the tendency for infectious organisms to develop resistance to antibiotics. One sibling asked, "What happens if someone else catches an infection from Daddy?" We explained that this does occur and creates difficult infections in other people. The family was horrified. They began an internal conversation about their father's commitment to helping others and to the concept of stewardship for natural resources.

One sister spoke up and said, "He would never have wanted this, and we all know it." The next question was "What can we do?" After a brief discussion about *The Active Management of Dying*, they were quite ready to withdraw further medical intervention and artificial nutrition. They prayed together, thanked us, and took their father home. We received a thank-you note a few weeks later, after he had passed.

This case demonstrated something mentioned before. These people already had an intrinsic sense of the realities of the situation; they just needed a bit of knowledge and guidance to put their thoughts into action. It also reinforced the value of having an identified spokesperson and family leader. Although it took a while, once someone took the leadership role, the family was able to move forward with the plan they already knew was appropriate.

—— CASE 4: MS. PINCHON ——

The previous cases dealt with patients who were already incapacitated at the time medical futility was declared. It is perhaps tougher, though no less appropriate, to discuss *The Active Management of Dying* with coherent people who have terminal diseases.

Ms. Pinchon was in her early fifties when we met. She had been a patient in our practice for some time but had not come in for routine exams or sick care in several years. By her account, she was a woman with a "hard past" (alcohol and IV drug use) who had turned her life around and was proud of her successful family of two generations. She had been "clean and sober" for over fifteen years, and watched over her adult children and adolescent grandchildren with a wizened viewpoint. She came in concerned about the yellowing of her face and eyes, which had been getting worse over the last few months. She also felt that her belly was swelling. She had obviously overcome some denial that she was sick, but was not happy to be in the office that day.

Her exam revealed a large, lumpy, slightly tender liver, and a fluid-filled abdomen. Lab tests proved that her liver was in serious trouble. I strongly suspected liver cancer and sent her across the street for a scan of her abdomen. Several hours later the result was back, and it was not good. Her liver was literally packed with tumors, and she had evidence of them spreading to several other areas. We sat together alone in an exam room, with her granddaughter and son outside.

"What is it, Doc?" she asked.

I was tempted to sugarcoat it, to make her feel better and hide behind my own denial. I liked this rugged, independent woman. "The scan shows a lot of densities in your liver and abdomen. Although we need a biopsy and other tests to confirm, I won't lie to you. It looks like cancer, and it is very advanced."

To my surprise she only chastised herself briefly for delaying the visit so long. Then she asked, "What do we do?"

I paused and said, "I think we should put you in the hospital over the weekend and monitor you. We can try to get the biopsy in the next couple of days, then discuss options."

"How long do I have?" she asked softly.

"I don't know, the tests will tell us more."

She thought for a bit, and then said, "If your liver is shot and the cancer is all over, they can't fix all that...I want to go home."

Although I could understand her point, as her doctor I had to inform her, "Ms. Pinchon, you are sick. Your liver is failing. It's leaking fluid into your abdomen, which will probably get infected, and it's not even making clotting factors for your blood. I am not sure you'll make it through the weekend at home."

She was not to be dismayed. She promised she would come back as an outpatient for her tests, but said she had personal and family work to do. She vowed she would not die in the hospital.

I could not blame her, nor could I find any reason to try to convince her to change her mind. She had not shown signs of mental illness or recent substance abuse prior to the findings. It was clear she had the capacity to make informed decisions, and her logic was difficult to dispute. Although I assumed she must have some emotional shock and denial, she remained in complete control. I could not promise her or myself that the hospital had much to offer her in this particular case, so I could not justify insisting we had a better option. Her family was invited in, and they were also unable to change her mind.

So, I said, "Ms. Pinchon, you must understand I have to recommend hospitalization for you. However, if you refuse, that is your right. I believe you understand that your disease could be fatal, even in a few days. I am torn because I don't want you to forgo some beneficial medical or surgical treatment, but I also do not want you to be in pain at home if things deteriorate rapidly. So, I would like to ask hospice to at least be aware of your case, that way if you need them they can help you. We can order the outpatient biopsy in the meantime."

I called the local hospice care provider and explained the situation. Although we were not declaring an end to all medical procedures, I told them I did feel she had a reasonable life expectancy of less than six months (a major criterion for hospice involvement). They understood the patient's position and agreed to come to the home if she needed them. At that point they would register her as a hospice patient and care for her comfort. She liked this plan. She went home and got much worse. It was clear that she had end-stage liver cancer. She died within twenty-four hours, but not before writing meaningful letters to each of her family members, typing out a brief will, and calling hospice for support and pain medicine. Her family grieved but spoke with respect about "Mom's stubbornness." They did request an autopsy to know for sure what had happened. It confirmed the CT scan results. Her abdomen and chest were riddled with metastatic tumors, originating from her liver, which was twice normal size.

Even though she would not have lived much longer, this was not a clear-cut case. In this case medical futility was strongly suspected, and the patient exercised her autonomy, against medical advice (although I silently cheered her tenacity and pragmatism as she rejected my advice). I have discussed this case with several colleagues. Most agree with the decisions. A few said they would not offer hospice if she refused medical advice, because of the liability risk to them and the overall principle of it. That position alarmed me greatly as it seemed too physician-centered rather than patient-centered. A few also felt I should have been more vague with the preliminary results to "buy some more time." Perhaps then she would have consented to hospitalization and tests. I can only say that it would have been regretful if her last days on Earth were filled with hospital paperwork and needle sticks, rather than writing those letters and making her peace. She asked for an honest opinion, and that is what she received. In any event, the decision was hers, and barring some reason to the contrary, it had to be respected. For more information about this subject, see Bert's discussion in Chapter 2, "Moral Decision-Making."

A Personal Note

Because this whole subject of death and dying is very personal and very sensitive I think it is proper to share my own personal experience with the reader because I think it will help you understand and realize our common humanity.

My grandmother, Pauline, was a sweet and loving grandmother to me. Throughout my childhood, she gave me breakfast in bed and bragged on me to everyone who knew her. This is the beauty of grandmothers. As she grew older, and I grew up, her health began to decline. I remember a vague awareness that she was slowly declining. I did not want to know it; I did not want to accept it. I wanted her to go out and hike in the woods with me when I was twenty-five years old just like she did when I was five. As she got older and in poorer states of health, she was not always as sweet and cheerful as she had been when I was younger. I did not want to accept that either. When she began to have chronic pain from severe osteoporosis (thinning of the bones), and the vertebral collapse that comes with it, her life became miserable.

I was actually in residency during this time and lived several hours away. It was always very difficult for me to know that I was taking care of people I hardly knew and was unable to take care of my beloved grandmother. Fortunately, her doctor was the father of a friend of mine, and I knew she was in good hands. Her husband, Sam, was very attentive, and my father moved near their home to be available.

As we watched her decline, our entire immediate family went through all the same stages and problems that most other families would. I remember experiencing and watching others experience denial, misplaced anger, fear, depression, pain, and a dread of acknowledging my own mortality. I witnessed arguments as well as compassionate discussions. I watched my grandfather's desperate attempts to find a miracle cure and the perfect doctor or hospital that could "fix" her.

As she became bed-bound, and in so much pain that she was on continuous narcotic medications, her doctor finally said to my grandfather, "Sam, she will never feel better until she is with God." It was the blatant honesty and lack of ambiguity of the statement that allowed my grandfather to gain acceptance. His focus changed because of this. He attended to her constantly, and his only goal was to keep her comfortable. He no longer fought the idea that she was going to die and leave him; his focus was simply on her needs at that time. This release from responsibility and guilt passed to the rest of us. The arguments stopped, the compassion increased, and Pauline suffered less. She stabilized for a while, but eventually her will to live waned. A few months later she died peacefully, in the home she'd occupied for over half a century, under the watchful care of hospice. We experienced grief and sadness, but we did not experience shock. It took several years for the family to recover once the matriarch had passed; however, healing did occur and life moved on.

I offer this to the reader for two reasons. First, when one deals frankly and firmly with death and dying, one can be construed as cold and unfeeling. This is far from the truth. What I learned is that by being firm and honest one can extend the greatest compassion to someone who is in the dying process. If one is overwhelmed by emotions such as anger, guilt, and denial, one may actually leave a loved one defenseless and vulnerable. I have no regrets about my grandmother's death. I know it was managed properly. While I wish we could have orchestrated her care a little sooner, I understood that the people involved had to come to their own acceptance before we could accomplish a good care plan. Obviously, I hope this book helps you along that path as well.

Notes

8

Specific Advice *for* End-of-Life Care

Lance writes...

For best understanding, it would be wise to read the advice for each group, even if it does not apply to you specifically. There is purposeful redundancy from previous chapters to reinforce the concepts.

For Patients

The following is my most honest and heartfelt advice for the person of sound mind who is facing a terminal disease, and for whom conventional medicine has nothing left to offer. This advice is distilled from my experience, readings and teachings I have received on the subject, and familiarity with the medical system and disease processes. I would go so far as to say these are "Doctor's orders."

1. Consider a second opinion and/or a repeat office visit with your doctor to make sure you completely understand all the information you've received about your health problem.

2. Find out how certain your doctor is about your prognosis. Ask tough questions and expect honest answers. You will need to feel sure that the condition is terminal and not curable. You will feel a furious rush of painful emotions. These are normal. Talk to your doctors, your religious leader, family, and friends. Do not be afraid to speak about your condition and ask for help. If you have multiple doctors involved in your care and are getting different individual opinions, insist on a face-to-face meeting with all of them present. Ask them to confront each other and come to a consensus about your best options. It is all too common that doctors will express differing opinions in the absence of their colleagues, and this is unfair to the layperson who is caught in the middle.

3. After a period of time, when you have gotten yourself together, hold a family meeting. If you have not filled out a living will and health care power of attorney (appropriate to your state), obtain those documents (they are free at **www.atthecloseofday.com**), and bring them to the meeting. Tell those present what is happening. Allow them to grieve and be shocked. Then, let them know you want to work on this problem with their support. Fill out the living will and health care power of attorney, and encourage those present to use this opportunity to do the same for themselves; you will all realize the importance of it. Ask your family to read this book or other similar literature to help them understand what you are doing. Appoint a health care power of attorney to be your spokesperson if you become unable to speak for yourself. Let your family know your wishes regarding end-of-life care. This will relieve them of much guilt and panic, and will help you be more comfortable. As you do this you will feel a sense of order and control over your situation, despite an uncontrollable disease.

4. Discuss hospice as an option. Let your doctor and family know you would like hospice care when the time becomes appropriate. Consider meeting with hospice representatives early and pick one you feel good about. Be cautious not to develop undue expectations of your hospice, however. They do wonderful work but are not without limits. Have honest communication about what you would like, and how much service they can provide.

5. Plan your legal will and estate early. You do not want to face legal battles in your final days.

6. Make spiritual peace in whatever form you need to. (See Bert's discussion above.) Inspire your loved ones by letting them know that work is ongoing. They will be forever reassured by your example, and you will be even more at peace in that knowledge. As you do your spiritual work, you will feel other areas of your life come into focus as well.

7. Discuss your funeral arrangements, including whether or not you wish to have a wake. Finishing this business will also give you greater peace and make room for more pleasant things.

8. Live. Live as fully as you can in your final days. No one can predict exactly how long any of us have, and you may completely disprove all of your doctors' opinions (doctors do love to be wrong sometimes). As you plan for a good death, live your life with unbridled passion. Plan trips and events you have dreamed about for years. Do not worry if you never get to finish them; remember that you might get to do them. Ask forgiveness, and give it to those people for whom you have had anger.

Eat well, exercise, and keep order in your life. This will give you your best chance for a longer, healthier existence. Say "I love you" whenever you can. Laugh whenever possible. Cry whenever necessary.

9. You do not have to live in pain. A good physician can work with you to find dosages of pain medication that allow you to be awake and comfortable at the same time, so that you can maximize your freedom, independence, and activities.

10. Give. Find a way to give back. Pass wisdom to a child. Make a gift to a cause you believe in. Take whatever steps are necessary to know that you have touched the world in a positive way.

11. Do not wait for death. Embrace the opportunity to live. Once you accept that your lifeline is shorter than you expected, the little things don't matter. (That piece of advice applies at any age, in any state of health.) Take chances you never would have taken. Laugh off the advice to "take it easy." You will know your limits.

For Families

If you have a family member who is dying or severely debilitated and getting worse, this section is for you. Be sure that you have read and absorbed all the above advice for patients. If you serve as the faithful accompanier (for the person who still has capacity) or the surrogate (if the person has lost capacity), you will find it useful.

1. Acknowledge that you are in a difficult situation. If you are the primary care giver or HCPOA/spokesperson, you may feel a tremendous sense of responsibility and angst. First, you must let some of it go. You must allow yourself to accept that you neither caused, nor can you change, this condition. All you can do is to help the loved one suffer as little as possible. Make sure your questions have been answered by the patient's doctor(s), and that you have asked very direct questions about prognosis and what to expect. Do not be afraid to get the doctors together for a consensus regarding options. If the patient still has the ability to make decisions, by all means let him, it is his life. But be ready to step in, if and when the situation mandates.

2. Understand the dying person's perspective. Speak with the patient at length about his wants and desires, and make sure you can carry them out, but do not be afraid to help him confront reality if he is in tremendous denial. Bert's excellent guidance above will serve you very well. Allow yourself to accept the powerful but limited nature of your role.

3. If you serve as the surrogate, assert yourself as the spokesperson and representative of the dying person. Make sure the rest of the family knows you have been named, or are acting as, spokesperson and decision-maker. Listen to their concerns and tell them yours, but be clear that once the patient has lost his decision-making ability you will be the final voice, and that you will act as the patient's advocate, according to what you heard from and know of the patient. Ask other family members to read this book or similar literature so you all can be on the same page. You are literally dealing with life and death issues. Ambiguity and indecision have no place, for the consequences are serious.

I will use a simplistic example to make a point, but please do not think I am minimizing the seriousness of the issue. Do you remember those two little cartoon rodents, I believe they were hedgehogs, who were so polite that they would each wait for the other to go first into a safe hole when the predator approached? They needed leadership and decisiveness during the crisis. During any emergency, be it war, natural disaster, fire, or medical crisis, chaos is the enemy. Without identified leaders, people will get hurt or killed unnecessarily. Dying is inherently chaotic, and the surrogate becomes the leader who shields the patient from chaos during his vulnerable time. This may mean advocating for more pain medicine, assuring that painful procedures are not performed against the patient's wishes (and that does happen far too often), or channeling family arguments away from the bedside.

You have become a leader. After the initial meetings and discussions ask everyone to run further questions and concerns through you to the doctor(s), and let the doctors know that is the plan. Nothing distracts a doctor from good care of a patient as much as trying to answer to several family members who have different opinions and questions. Do not be afraid to delegate and consult. Leave legal matters to lawyers. Get hospice and home services in early. Your mission is clear and of utmost importance...helping your loved one to achieve a good death.

Do not let health care professionals convince you to do things against the wishes of the patient. If the patient said he would never want to be kept alive on tubes and lines, then hold to that, and tell everyone that it is not your wish...it is the patient's.

4. Release guilt and fear. If you feel tempted to utilize medical interventions in a terminally ill person, ask yourself, "Who am I trying to help, me or my loved one?" If the person is unable to get out of bed or communicate, is lying on bedsores in his own excrement, and will not take enough food or fluid to sustain life, and you decide on a feeding tube to prolong that situation indefinitely, it may be that you are serving your own guilt rather than the person's best interest. It is all right to let go of that. Again, you did not invent death and disease, nor can you ultimately stop it.

5. Be proud of your role and of your service. When your loved one does die, know that you have done everything you could to make it a comfortable passage for him. A side of you may feel relieved when it is over. This is very normal and you are not obligated to feel guilty for that relief. You will have just completed one of the most difficult of tasks. You deserve a vacation and a medal, not a guilt trip or remorse. Consider it a victory that your loved one died well, and you helped to achieve that. Acknowledge that the alternatives would have been much worse. You may have come close to breaking at many points, but you did not. You may feel you could have done it better. You probably could not have. You passed the test. You did your job.

If your job were to build a beautiful house, and you did so, would you feel guilty when it was completed? Of course not! You would feel proud and relieved. So if you are the spokesperson for a dying person, your job is to help him achieve as close to an ideal death as possible. It is not to make him live longer, much less forever. The doctors could not even do that. Therefore, when he dies as comfortably as possible, consider it a job well done. You will need to grieve, but you will never need to feel guilty. This lesson is universal and it is as difficult for doctors to accept as anyone else, but once it is accepted, the entire dying process can be viewed in a completely different and much more tolerable fashion.

For Health Care Professionals

The next section is dedicated to health care professionals, especially medical students and physicians-in-training (residents) who have questions and fears about managing the dying process. This section has value to the layperson as well because it will help to illustrate how the health care professional must think about such cases. These points are integral to *The Active Management of Dying.*

To my current and future colleagues, I implore you to take this topic very seriously. We are well aware that our nursing homes are full of people who have lived far beyond their natural years to questionable benefit. It breaks our hearts when we see someone who is bed-bound, contracted, and riddled with bedsores. We feel a certain angst when we treat a recurrent pneumonia or urinary tract infection in a completely bed-bound person, knowing full well that the infection will be back within a few weeks or a month, and it will get worse each time. My feeling is that, by employing techniques of *The Active Management of Dying*, we can help avoid the unfortunate situation where the patient lives indefinitely in a state of suffering, well past the point of medical futility.

The other benefit is that it allows us all to avoid the highly controversial issue of euthanasia. Our individual beliefs on that subject are varied, but if we all focus on what we *can* do for the dying, I believe it will be a win-win situation for all participants, and our efforts will be united. That has been my experience when I have employed the techniques as described above. I wish you well in your attempts to *actively manage* the dying process to the benefit of the patient.

Go ahead and imagine that you have been presented with a patient, Mrs. Brown, who has been ill for some time. Perhaps she is demented or has had several strokes. The clinical course has deteriorated recently. She is failing to thrive, she is not taking sufficient food and/or fluid to sustain life, and everyone is aware that things are not improving.

1. **Assess the patient**. Of course this sounds simple, but what I mean by this is *really* assess the patient. Examine the patient alone, just you and the patient. Then review the chart. Find out what has happened and familiarize yourself with the case to date, as you would with any patient. Before you tell the family anything, talk with them, and find out what the clinical course has been. After the patient and family have

helped you understand the events leading to your contact with them, help them see the evolution of this disease and dying process. When applicable, have them describe when their loved one lost the ability to communicate or care for herself. Have them explain how many infections, how many emergency room visits, and how many hospitalizations have occurred. They will trust you because you are concerned enough to dig deeper than a superficial history. They will also illustrate to themselves the reality and gravity of the situation. Find out who the patient was before she began to deteriorate. Ask the family "How did she live her life? What were her beliefs?" Ask the family how it felt to watch this person, who was once vigorous, slide into a state where she could no longer care for herself.

2. Offer human interaction to the family. Sit down with them, talk to them, person-to-person, on a human level, and just find out information. Offer to buy them a cup of coffee. They will be tired, and your simple kindness will go a long way. They have probably been keeping a vigil over this situation for some time. They have probably shed many tears and had arguments and fights over the situation. Of course, if the patient *can* communicate with you in any form, talk to her, both one-on-one, in a quiet setting, as well as in front of the family. Let the family and the patient know that your focus is on the patient, but the family's health and wishes are also your concern.

3. Identify a spokesperson. Do this early, and if the family has not already done so, leave them for a while and ask them to identify the spokesperson. You will find it very difficult if you try to speak to several family members at once. Once the spokesperson is identified, begin directing the conversation to that person. Obviously, you do not want to be rude or exclude other family members, but make it clear that the spokesperson must be the channel for all their concerns, questions, and anxieties. You simply must be focused and productive in this regard, or you will not be able to help the patient as well as you might. Keep your mind on your goal: *helping the patient.* Reiterate that whenever the conversation loses focus. Family members may feel the need to branch off into other issues, but you will need to bring the focus back to the painful reality of the patient's declining status.

4. Step back and look at your data and reactions objectively. After you've gathered your information, done your exam, and gotten understanding of the dynamics of the family, take a moment. Consider the following questions: Is there anything else that modern medicine has to offer this patient in terms of cure or therapy? Is there any real point to prolonging life or suffering? In other words, is this patient dying? If so, focus again on your goal—to help your patient die as comfortably and peacefully as possible. Reflect on your own feelings. If you feel you will be failing in your role as a physician by "letting" this patient die, you will have difficulty in this situation. If you can readjust your mindset to accept that there is much you can do for the dying patient, and this is part of your role as physician, you will stand to make a tremendous difference in the patient's life as well as the life of the family. Consider the idea that death can be a peaceful outcome of good care, rather than any sort of failure.

5. Reflect on the practical and logistical steps it will take to accomplish your goal. What paperwork will be required to make sure your treatment plan is carried out as seamlessly as possible? How will the family respond to your diagnosis and prognosis, and how can you help them accept a reality they may not want to hear? Be ready to summon personnel from the hospital and your practice to help you. This may include nurses, social workers, and clergy, as well as disposition managers, nurse managers, and ethics committee members. In most states, medical futility can be declared by the consistent opinion of two licensed physicians. It would be a good idea to know of a trusted colleague who would not hesitate to reevaluate your diagnosis and prognosis if needed.

6. Be ready to approach the family with the diagnosis and prognosis, once you have the logistical plan in your head. Sit them down in a room, with the spokesperson closest to you. Offer them comfort and refreshments if needed. Let them know you have carefully examined their loved one, reviewed the chart, and considered what you and they know about the patient. Reiterate that your concern is primarily the patient's comfort. Be frank and firm with your language. The family is now looking to you as an authority. They may not like everything you have to say, but your opinion does carry weight. Be very careful *not* to make statements unless you are confident in their certainty. For example, you may be very strong in the opinion that further medical intervention is futile for the patient and comfort measure are appropriate, but you may not know how long this patient has to live. It would sabotage the family's trust of you if you made predictions that were grossly incorrect. A sample conversation may go as follows:

> *"Hello again, everyone. I'm Doctor Smith. I've met some of you, and we have talked; others, I am glad to meet you. I have reviewed Mrs. Brown's case history and examined her thoroughly. I had a good conversation with the rest of the family, and I think I have an understanding of what many of her wishes would be in this situation. I want you to understand that my purpose here is to act in the best interests of Mrs. Brown.*

"It is clear to me that she has been in declining health for some time. It is also clear to me that things have gotten much worse lately. I think you probably have a sense that she is not getting better. You have noticed an increase in hospital visits and infections. She obviously eats and drinks very little. These are all very clear signs that she is now in the dying process. In my professional opinion, I do not feel we have any medical intervention that would be of benefit to her. I don't think any artificial life-prolonging measures, including breathing tubes, feeding tubes, or artificial fluids, would do anything but prolong her suffering. I also feel that treating infections would do nothing but prolong her suffering.

"However, I think there are many things we *can* do on her behalf. I think we can make her much more comfortable than she is now. We can do this with medications and increased care. I think that bringing hospice into the home would help by keeping her in familiar surroundings. Her home is much better than the chaotic emergency room, where she may feel some sense of fear. I want to keep her from being stuck with needles and lines unnecessarily because we do not want to cause her pain. We can use medications to keep her from having seizures or other problems. We can apply mouth care so she doesn't feel thirsty or have cracked lips. We can arrange for emotional and spiritual support for both her and the rest of the family. If any of the family members are having trouble with sleeping or nervousness, I would be happy to see you as patients and try to help you with these problems."

After such a statement, you will find that most families are ready to accept your prognosis of the dying process, but may yet be riddled with guilt.

7. Address the guilt issues. I have found tremendous power in the following language: "I have managed patients in this state many times. After examining and hearing about her, it is clear to me that she is in the dying process, and further medical intervention is futile. You have been carrying a heavy burden for a long time, and the decisions we are talking about are very difficult and carry much guilt. That time is over for you now. You are relieved of that burden. My plan now is to move forward with comfort measures, making sure your loved one is as well cared for as possible and you have more services in the home to help with this process. In other words, as her doctor, I am taking the responsibility out of your hands."

As you become comfortable with this style of language, you will begin to experience a wonderful phenomenon as patients and families realize the release you are offering. Be aware, however, that some families will not accept this, and will want you to order tests and treatments and procedures that you do not feel are appropriate. It is important for you to understand that legally you are not obligated to perform medical interventions that you feel are not in the patient's best interests. If the family cannot accept your prognosis, diagnosis, and plan, you have the option of withdrawing from the case and finding another physician for the patient. The next physician may also agree with your assessment and plan, and eventually this will help the family to accept reality. It is possible the next physician may have a different approach, and the family may like this better. In any event, you will have had the opportunity to stand on your principles and offer your best advice. If the patient or family is having trouble accepting your words, offer to step out of the room, and let them talk among themselves prior to making a decision or statement. Again, remind them you would like the designated spokesperson or health care power of attorney to have the final say in the matter.

You may find that initially these conversations are very awkward for you. I would consider that a normal reaction. You may blush, feel guilty, stutter, and have other obviously anxious reactions. It would be wise to practice your dialogue prior to meeting with families; just like any actor, you can avoid some of your stage fright. Patients and families will need your professional objectivity and your confidence, even if you are feeling very human inside. After you have been through *The Active Management of Dying* process several times, this will feel as comfortable to you as any other part of your medical practice.

8. Tie it all together. Let's now assume that you've had your meeting with the family, it is accepted that the patient is dying, and they realize that further medical intervention is futile. Comfort measures are the appropriate next step. If the patient was not well enough to be part of that decision, make a visit to the bedside. Even if the patient has no evidence of awareness or interaction, it will do you well to go through the ceremony of telling the patient what you are going to do for her. For example, "Mrs. Brown, this is Doctor Smith. I want you to know I understand that you may be uncomfortable. I want you to know we are going to do everything we can to make you more comfortable, and we will make sure that your needs are looked after. Your family is planning to be with you, and the nursing staff and I will also be caring for you." This simple act may have immense value to the patient whose consciousness is not as low as suspected. It will certainly help complete the process for you, and it will comfort the family enormously.

9. Coordinate with other professionals. The next step would be to notify any other health care workers involved with the patient about the plan. This would include consulting physicians, nursing staff, nursing home staff, any home health agencies or workers, and any hospice agencies or workers who are already involved. Make it very clear to them that the patient, family, and you, as the physician, have decided the patient is terminal and medical intervention is futile. Tell them you are moving toward the comfort care model. Recruit them to support the decision. Help them understand that further trips to the hospital or resuscitative, life-prolonging measures are against the plan. Help them to be comfortable that if the patient were to die while they were in attendance, that this would be a satisfactory outcome. Without confidence, other professionals involved in the care may panic or lose focus at crucial moments, and may disrupt even the most well designed plans. I cannot stress enough how important this communication is to the care of the dying. Understand that a nurse or nurse's aide may have no idea of the plan, and feel that they are doing the right thing by calling 911, as the patient is about to die. For the patient's benefit, you must be very thorough at this step. Stay keenly aware of the potential for conflicting opinions and views among other health care providers. Communicate frequently among other team members and hold meetings with everyone present if at all possible. Try to round at the same time as other consultants so that the patient and family see a unified team.

10. Documentation. The next step is logistical. Dictate or write a note in the patient's chart describing your assessment of the patient's condition, your meeting with the family, who was in attendance, and pertinent items discussed. Finish the note with your impression of the terminal and medically futile status of the patient. Then, describe your treatment plan, which again would be to provide comfort, palliative and/or hospice care, whether in the home, nursing home or hospital environment. You will then need to obtain a hospital Do Not Resuscitate order form. Put this on the chart after writing "Do Not Resuscitate" on the routine order page. You will probably also want to adjust your treatment plan by writing orders to stop tube feedings and intravenous hydration, liberal orders for pain control and anti seizure medications, and orders for mouth care. Often a hospice or social work consult is indicated at this time. (See Appendix B for sample orders.)

11. Anticipate other confounders. Keep in mind that many states require a separate Do Not Resuscitate order to be placed at the patient's bedside, if the patient is away from the hospital, specifically for emergency medical service personnel. If the patient is returning to a nursing home, you will need to rewrite the comfort care orders of the hospital, and, even if hospice will be involved, you will want to write initial orders for pain control. I have also written orders such as "Do not treat with antibiotics, "Do not transport," and "No artificial hydration or nutrition," to prevent confusion. Also be aware that most states expect the doctor to be knowledgeable about the Out-of-Hospital DNR and that it is stocked in the doctor's office.

12. Appreciate your planning. Realize that the investment that you make early in this process will facilitate a much smoother death for the patient with less angst on your part, the patient's part and the family's part. If you omit steps in the planning, you may see a breakdown of your management. Your patient, who could have died peacefully at home, may end up back at the emergency room, even without your knowledge. Keep in mind that "the system" is *never* perfect, and in this regard, you are protecting your patient from the default pathway, which is chaos and sub-optimal care. The default pathway is essentially that "all people must be resuscitated whenever possible unless these matters have been clarified in advance." You are trying to orchestrate a more elegant process.

13. Arrange for the patient to be in the best possible environment. Once all these concerns have been addressed, if your patient is in the hospital you will realize there is no need for further hospitalization. The family should be aware that you are planning to discharge the patient from the hospital in relatively short order, but that you would like to give them time to prepare the home environment if the patient will be returning there. Often a hospice representative can meet with the family in the hospital prior to discharge to facilitate this, or less ideally, the hospice representative can go to the home shortly after discharge. This will comfort the family tremendously, and facilitate the transfer. Give the family specific instructions for common scenarios; for example, help them to understand that they do not have to dial 911 anymore, that it is all right if the patient actually dies at home. They may still be unclear on this point. If hospice is in place, a worker will be a phone call away and can help with these concerns.

14. Consider care for the family. It is advisable to go ahead and make a follow-up appointment for the patient's family to meet with you, within a day or two of discharge, so they know they can talk to someone. This will alleviate many anxious feelings. At that time you can do an assessment for problems of insomnia or undue emotional trouble.

15. Other techniques. I have found a few simple techniques that help to reassure the family and relieve guilt even further. The first of these is to go ahead and let the family offer or assist with food and fluid by mouth. Just because artificial food and hydration is gone, does not mean that the patient is unable to take food and fluid naturally. Remember, *The Active Management of Dying* is about a natural process, not euthanasia, and there is no reason to prevent feeding if the patient can accept it by natural routes. Many clinicians have expressed concern over possibility of aspiration (inhaling food or fluid) if a debilitated person is fed. It is important to remember that we are talking about a stage of the dying process where aspiration or aspiration pneumonia will hasten death a little, but that is all right. It is still a natural part of the dying process. The family may feel great reassurance that they are offering food, even if the patient decides to refuse or cannot participate in the feeding process.

I once encountered an interesting scenario in which a family acknowledged futility and wanted to take their loved one home to die in her bed. The immediate family was very comfortable with the decision, but they didn't want to have to explain the decision to distant family, friends and other visitors. Therefore, they asked if we could provide an IV pole and a bag of fluids to drip slowly in to the patient's vein. I started to explain that we did not want to hydrate the patient, and they understood that. The goal was not to hydrate the patient, but to simply give the illusion that there was some medical intervention occurring. We set the rate at one drip every two minutes, which would have no clinical significance, but apparently had great symbolic significance to the visitors, and the family felt very reassured that they would not be questioned as to their care of the dying patient. We found this relatively easy to arrange, and this basically completed the negotiations. The point to all this is that each person may have different beliefs, values and cultural concerns. By working with the family, and keeping an open mind, much can be accomplished in short order.

Dementia

I want to give special attention to the condition of dementia, as it is probably very confusing to the layperson. Dementia essentially refers to a long-term state of decreased cognitive (mental) ability. In other words, a person doesn't think, reason, or function as well as he once did. Alzheimer's disease is the best known example.

Dementia has a variety of causes. A stroke, or several strokes, can starve parts of the brain of oxygen, and those parts are permanently damaged. When several parts of the brain have been affected, the overall brain cannot function as well, and we call this multi-infarct (multi-stroke) dementia. Alzheimer's disease is a generalized loss of nerve function in the brain, and we are not entirely sure why it happens. It appears to be a combination of genetic, environmental, and intrinsic factors. Toxicity, such as prolonged alcohol abuse and other exposure to poisons and drugs, can also result in progressive dementia. Nutritional deficiencies, untreated syphilis, or a long history of mental illness may also cause dementia.

An afflicted person will progressively lose parts of his memory. Often the short and intermediate memories are lost first. As more and more memories and cognitive (thinking) function are lost, people with dementia may become unable to care for themselves. They are at risk to hurt themselves on normal household objects. They may roam aimlessly about inside and outside of their homes. They may become unpleasant as different aspects of the personality become uninhibited. They may eventually lose control of their bodily functions as the part of the brain that keeps people aware of these no longer functions properly. Over time, profoundly demented people will be bed-bound and will neglect even the most basic activities of living, such as eating and drinking. Although we do not always think of dementia as a terminal disease, it certainly can become one.

Most forms of dementia are irreversible, although there are certain medications and therapies that can delay their progression. To a demented person, familiar surroundings such as home and photographs are generally comforting, but new surroundings may be terrifying. Imagine you woke up with an almost empty mind, not remembering who or where you are. If you looked around to see comfortable surroundings, such as a bed or photographs that at one time had meaning to you, there is a chance that these would comfort you. However, a chaotic and alienated environment, such as an emergency room or a hospital, could be a terrifying experience. This is an important consideration when you are determining the best treatment plan for a chronically demented person. Ideally you would want to keep him at home and comfortable rather than frequently transported or changing environments.

Notes

9

Grieving

"Sweeping Up the Heart and Putting Love Away"

Bert writes . . .

Emily Dickinson, grief's eloquent apprentice, wrote this poem in 1866: [7]

> The Bustle in a House
> The Morning after Death
> Is solemnest of industries
> Enacted upon Earth—
>
> The Sweeping up the Heart
> And putting Love away
> we shall not want to use again
> Until Eternity.

When my father-in-law died, they were sitting around the kitchen table the next morning and his wife or one of his daughters remembered that poem. She brought out the old volume of Emily Dickinson's poems and

---

[7] *First Harvest: Emily Dickinson's Poems*, Poem 415 (Boston: Little, Brown & Company, 1961).

read it aloud. They shared the silence together for a moment before getting busy with all the bustle of things that have to be done "the morning after death." I wonder if, in that moment, they weren't glancing ahead to the days of sorrow and nights of loneliness before them in the path of mourning, drawing from the poem an unforgettable image to help them through.

I love that metaphor. Grieving is a "sweeping up the heart/and putting love away." Not that it is tidy. Grieving is messy and very hard work, taking its toll both physically and emotionally. It doesn't fit into neat stages. Sometimes it seems to crawl forward and then loop back on itself, reliving the same memories, relearning the same lessons, feeling again the same pain. If grief is like sweeping, then the same piece of the heart's floor must be swept again and again, as grief takes all the time it needs to put love away in a safe place. Grief takes its own time, and in our rush to return to a routine, or just to feel better again, we sometimes try to brush the slow work of grieving aside. But until grief's work is done, brushing it aside only prolongs its duration.

What is grief's work, and why does it take so long? A friend told it this way: "Imagine how swiftly death comes upon us. A judge's gavel dismisses a twenty-year marriage in a second. A surgeon removes a breast or a limb in one tight morning's schedule. A fetus is aborted...a moving van pulls away from a lifelong home...a loved one is alive one moment and, with a breath, is utterly gone. How can we possibly absorb the shattering devastation of that loss in such an instant? Grief comes to carry the past with us until we have made it our own, until we are grounded in it and have made meaning of it and can slowly, piece by agonizing piece, let it go. Phillips Brooks wrote in a letter to a friend whose mother had recently died: 'People bring us well meant but miserable consolations when they tell us what time will do to help our grief. We do not want to lose our grief, because our grief is bound up with our love, and we could not cease to mourn without being robbed of our affections.'" [8]

This, then, is what grief does: it grasps hold of the person who is gone, and holds him or her in our memory until we can fully understand and internalize all our experience with him, making him fully ours, so that when we are ready we can then release and let go what is past, or "put love away."

Grief work is basically memory work. We remember our loved one in a thousand ways: we tell the stories, walk around in the rooms, sit at the familiar table, let our imaginations relive scenes we have shared; and we *feel intensely all the feelings* embedded in these memories. Some memories are full of joy, and we feel corresponding sorrow in realizing their times are beyond our recovery. Some memories may bring remorse, anxiety, or even anger at the loved one or at ourselves. Memories come back laden with emotion. That's why grief is not *an* emotion but a wide and wild range of emotions—sadness, fear, anger, relief, guilt, yearning, anguish, and many more—and that's why grieving is such hard work. These feelings are heavy, and we have to carry them all alone.

My friend said, "Grief insists on its truth, its pain, its tears. Grief does not want to be consoled. How often we think that the loving thing to do is to somehow lessen the grief of one we care about by comforting them with our religious beliefs. While the words of the Bible and the promises of our faith are true, grief cannot hear them. The reality of grief is the absence of God and the "sounds of silence" needing to be acknowledged. The only consolation for grief is the gift of a friend who wants only to hold my hand, to be not profound but simply present, to be broken-hearted in my pain."

Grief takes us all the way to the bottom of our pain by evoking memories both fresh and long-forgotten. As much as we feel we want to, we should never try to take this pain away from one who is grieving, even when it seems unbearable, by shielding the person from his or her

---

[8] Susan H. Muesse, unpublished paper.

memories. "Don't think about it" is a mistake, whether given as advice or as a drug. Or if we ourselves are in grief's way, as much as we want out of the sadness, the weird mind-tricks, the depression, to be happy and feel ourselves again, we cannot get through with grief until grief is through with us.

Gradually—and this is the healing quality of grief—we are able to revisit the memories with a lessening of emotion. And then eventually, in grief's time, we can remember and speak of the loved one without weeping. That doesn't mean we have stopped loving him or her. It does mean that grief has done its healing work of putting love away without taking it away from us. Thus, grief allows us to experience the adventure of life again as whole persons, able to take on new challenges and new relationships. Perhaps we might even dare to enter into a relationship of the same kind that brought us such pain before.

Grief, then, as unwanted and painful and achingly slow as it can be, is *good*. It is a gift to help us through devastating loss. It can't change our loss—nothing can do that—but it can teach us how to survive our loss and recover our selfhood. Grief is an honest teacher, and grief's lesson to us is *how to sorrow*. We're always at risk of getting trapped in self-pity or depression and staying there. But mourning is something we can do with an inner guide that moves us beyond anger and self-pity into our true suffering, a precious part of our life we may never have lived in before. And then we may be led through our suffering into a wisdom and compassion, first for ourselves and then for others, deeper than we have ever known.

I believe this because I have experienced grief this way, and I have listened to others share their losses and have borne witness to their recovery. I don't think of grief as merely a subjective response to loss or the threat of loss. Grief seems to me to have a life and integrity of its own. It works within us its wisdom and healing when we walk with it; it holds onto us until we have completed its process and some new life emerges in us. Grief will lead us to peace but knows no shortcuts. There is no other way but through the forest of memories and no other guide but grief.

So what can we do? If grief is a friend and guide, how can we handle our grief so it can work best with us and bring us peace and healing? In other words, how can we pick up the broken pieces of our life and bring them together in a new wholeness?

I will describe *three tasks* for the person who is grieving the loss of a loved one.

The first task is for you to *get a clear understanding of what happened when the painful loss occurred.* Don't be afraid to ask the doctors and nurses to tell you what they have done for your loved one, how they managed his care, what decisions were made and why, so that you can get a clear picture of the death. You will probably experience an inner craving to know these things, and you will ask a dozen questions. Getting the picture clear is good because it helps memory work. Then, telling the story to someone else is a way of testing and finally accepting the reality of your loved one's death, and you may do this a hundred times over. Ask the questions and tell the story—you are helping grief do its work.

This is a good place to introduce the concept of the *healing of memory.* There may be certain memories that cause intense pain or guilt or remorse, and those memories sometimes play like a relentless tape in our heads, especially at night. There may be a scene that has seared into our mind like a hot iron and keeps coming back, causing us to feel anxiety or stress. How can memories such as these be healed and released, so that we can find peace?

I remember Sandra, a loving single parent whose son had cystic fibrosis. Three weeks after his death at age sixteen, she told me she relived his death every night and couldn't sleep, that she was utterly fatigued all the time. There seemed to be something in the scene of his death itself that was upsetting her. I asked her to tell me the story just like she relived it in her mind.

She said her son, Kevin, had had a recurring dream for many years. They called it the "black lion" dream. There was a fearful lion that would attack, but Kevin had the strength to throw it all the way to China. Toward the end, he only had the strength to throw it into the back yard, and then when he turned around there it would be again. It was terrifying.

The night before he died, Sandra talked to Kevin a long time about dying and the promises of scripture, as the family shared a strong religious faith. Kevin, she said, was loving and gentle as always, but worried that God might be angry with him because he couldn't do anything for God. She reassured him that it wasn't like that. She gave him the image of Jesus himself welcoming him to heaven. But the next night her son was beside himself with anxiety. He woke in the middle of the night cursing and thrashing, using foul, blasphemous language that horrified her. "It's coming, it's gross, it's here, I can't keep it away!" He was screaming again in the emergency room, and Sandra stayed outside, trembling with the horror, while a friend held her. Kevin died a few hours later.

Sandra was tormented by the scene of his final agony. She felt both guilt and shame for not staying with her son in the emergency room. Thankfully, most of us have much gentler, more graceful memories of the death of our loved one, and we can handle more easily the emotion they cause, which is usually deep but tender sadness. But Sandra needed healing of a different kind because when she visualized the scene, which she couldn't help doing every night, it was very negative.

I made a suggestion to Sandra. I asked her to notice when the memory stream began, like a tape playing inside her head. I suggested that when the tape began, she should *pray* the memories, addressing every detail of the memory stream to God, and asking God to cleanse and heal the memory. Her memory of that night would become like a visual narrative that was offered to God, every detail of it, for healing.

Neither I nor anyone else could "preach" to Sandra that she shouldn't feel guilt about not being with her son at the last or about not being able to replace his terrifying vision of the lion with a peaceful vision of Jesus. But as she practiced transforming the memory stream into a prayer each time it started up, she began to feel herself forgiven. She let herself realize she had done the best she could, and her shame melted away. Perhaps the technique of *praying* her memories of that night—addressing them to God and leaving them with God—also helped her to soften their jagged edges and to remember Kevin in ways that were positive, loving, and peaceful. If so, that is an example of the healing of memories. Normally, in grief, memories heal us. Sometimes, however, we need to take the initiative to heal them.

To summarize, it helps to get a clear picture of all that has happened, so we can "true up" memories and tell the stories in detail, with no letter from our unconscious left unopened and no scene hidden. Memory work heals.

The second task in helping grief do its work is to *keep your heart open to all the feelings that memories bring to the surface.* Let them all come to your full awareness. Name them, even the hurtful ones such as anger or guilt. During the first few weeks after the death, you will probably feel a physical need to weep out loud. Some mourners find themselves crying for hours at a time multiple times a day. Give yourself the time and privacy you need to open your heart to the weeping. Accept it, and accept yourself.

Later, people often find that the need to cry settles into a deep depression. The emotions are not as close to the surface but may become more complex, and they may make us feel crazy. It's not uncommon, for example, to lose concentration, be unable to make decisions, have bodily symptoms like the deceased had, forget about eating, be tired all the time but unable to sleep soundly, feel tightness of the throat or heaviness in the chest, have mood changes over the slightest things, or feel like you're experiencing life from the bottom of a well. This can go on for months, and becomes frightening, especially to people who are accustomed to being in control of themselves. Acknowledge that fear, if it comes up, and try to untangle the other feelings within your depression. If they are confusing, be aware of the feeling of confusion.

When I was grieving my father's death many years ago, there came a point about three months after he died when I panicked because I thought I was losing my mind. I couldn't enjoy life, or make simple decisions, or even think straight, and I had been stuck there for months. The acute feeling of panic lasted several days. That may have been the turning point in my grieving process. It literally scared me out of my depression—the panic itself injected the energy I needed to move on. When the panic cleared, I became aware of the feeling that I had turned a corner and was now on the pathway to wholeness, even if I still had a ways to go. To acknowledge that feeling is in itself liberating. It gives hope.

To keep the heart open to all the feelings memory brings to the surface means more than simply *acknowledging* them, although that's where it begins. And for some of us—men especially—who aren't fluent in the language of feelings, that is a big first step. Open-heartedness, though, also means *accepting* our feelings, and *loving* them, even when they cause us suffering. It's amazing to me that human beings have the capacity not only to feel but to stand back mentally from our feelings and consciously draw them down into the heart, where thought and feeling become one. Grief helps us to do that more than any other human process I know. When we let it happen, our inner life grows into peace and a greater measure of wisdom and compassion than we have known before.

The third task of grieving is to *transform the relationship from a physical one into one of memory, or one of a spiritual nature.* I am indebted to a wonderful grief counselor, Marion Blackshear, for this language. At a deep level, she says, we must accept that death and loss make irrevocable physical changes. Reality is different now; the loved person is no longer physically present with us. But that does not mean we forget who has died or what has been lost. "Special people are part of who we are forever," she says. "Often in an even more meaningful way as their internalized value becomes a part of moving ahead with our lives."[9] That means transforming the relationship from the physical to the spiritual, from the outer life to the inner life.

Just as I was writing the paragraph above, I spoke by phone with a dear friend who lost her husband exactly ten years ago. Their son, who bears a striking resemblance to his father both in appearance and manner, just had the first grandchild. It was a wonderful and joyful event for her, but the conjunction of the anniversary of the death and seeing her son in the role of new father, a role in which she had loved her husband, made the cup of memories overflow. For days she was in tears and acute anxiety. At first she thought she must not have grieved her husband at the time of his death because her feelings now seemed so fresh and overwhelming. Some of her memories, which she shared with me, made her feel the agony of guilt for not expressing her love well enough to him before he died. Mostly she felt profound sadness and loss. The intensity of her feelings was unexpected and frightened her. She even told her new husband she was not sure she could continue to be with him.

I had been there ten years ago when her husband died. I perceived their relationship during the last months of his life as one of amazing love and communication, and I remembered that they themselves had expressed how "completely married" they had become, more so than in

---

[9] Marion Blackshear, "Grief Information Packet," unpublished.

all their twenty-five previous years. On the phone, I told her my version of the story and gave evidence. (It is absolutely normal to experience moral anxiety or guilt in grieving, so much so that we often feel *false* guilt that can and should be corrected.) It may seem audacious, but I corrected her story. This was validated when she accepted what I said and quietly thanked me.

One important aspect of transforming a physical into a spiritual relationship is *truing up the story*. We find the *meaning*—the "internalized value" of the person and whatever learning and personal growth we experience through the loss—only when the story our memory speaks to us is true. Sharing our memories with others gives them the opportunity to help us get the story more true and internalize it.

Then another aspect of transforming the relationship into a spiritual one occurred in our conversation. My friend said that her husband had often "spoken" to her through the last ten years, and this had helped keep her steady in making choices. She didn't mean that she heard a physical voice (although that sometimes happens early in the grief process, when we haven't accepted that the loved one is gone). She meant, I think, that *who her husband was to her* continued to be part of her life in a meaningful way. His values, his firm way of making decisions, were so real to her that it was almost as though he were speaking still. I think that is healthy. I encouraged her to listen now to what he was saying to her, especially about the new grandbaby, and respond to him from out of her own feelings.

Under some circumstances, that could be poor counsel and lead to irrational behavior. I was confident enough, though, in the health of my friend's grieving process and her soundness of mind and spirit, to believe that such an internal conversation could only be a source of healing and peace. That is what I mean by transforming the relationship from a physical to a spiritual plane. Even after ten years, half of them spent in another mutually satisfying marriage, grief is walking with her still, guiding her through a rough time to a more complete resolution. Her continued love for her deceased husband should not be seen as taking away from her present relationship. She is finishing the long task of transforming her former physical relationship into a spiritual one—so that she can embrace physical life today in all its goodness. Could we not express that truth in a more poetic way? . . .

> The Sweeping up the Heart
> And putting Love away
> We shall not want to use again
> Until Eternity.

Lance writes . . .

Bert has given us a valuable roadmap for healing after the loss of a loved one. I would simply like to add some practical advice for grieving people, and to the health care providers watching out for them.

I do not believe that normal grieving should be medicated with antidepressants or sedatives. Indeed, those drugs may allow one to avoid dealing with the reality of the loss. This may in turn prevent one from moving through the proper stages of grieving and delay emotional healing. One should not expect to suffer a loss and feel no emotional pain. One should expect that the pain will eventually subside and healing will occur. There may be a role for psychiatric medications in those with *abnormal* grieving (prolonged or overly intense grief, substance abuse problems, or pre-existing mental illness), but this should be carefully evaluated with the grieving person's primary care physician and/or mental health professional. I would much rather see patients receive counseling and social support instead of pills.

However, I firmly believe that sleep deprivation can be a devastating and unnecessary consequence of a death in a family, and have seen it in many people who were coping well otherwise. Sleep-deprived people lose perspective and may have much more intense emotional reactions than they would if they were rested. They may experience physical pain and symptoms that will confuse and frighten them. We do not want appropriate grieving to be jeopardized by undue exhaustion. We want to support healthy grieving.

When I work with family members who have recently suffered loss, I ask them how they are sleeping and if they anticipate any problems sleeping. I try to always offer a reasonable supply (one to two weeks) of mild prescription sleeping medications to treat or prevent sleep deprivation. If I was the doctor for the person who died, I will prescribe a short supply for immediate family members even if they are not "officially" my patients. The newer sleeping pills are not very addicting and usually do not produce a "hangover," but any extended prescriptions should be monitored by the person's doctor. Of course, many people do not need or want sleeping aids, but if the doctor offers them, it spurs thinking about the issue. Usually, any need for sleeping aids is short-lived and people who are grieving appropriately notice a deeper, more restful sleep after one to two weeks.

I encourage the family members to see their own doctors within a week after a major loss, so they will know there is a place to go if depression or sleep disturbance get out of control, and so that an objective professional can look for any concerning signs. Often the act of visiting one's doctor and being reassured that one is grieving normally has a powerful therapeutic effect that can prevent emotional complications.

After Death Has Occurred

Lance writes . . .

Many people express anxiety about the events that will unfold once a person has died. There are concerns over funeral home selection, funeral arrangements, and estate issues. If the person dies at home, there may be increased concerns over proper management of the body and the bedclothes.

The best thing to say here is that it will work out. It simply will. Every community has systems in place to deal with these issues. The best way to help it work out and avoid anxiety and confusion is to follow the same principle emphasized throughout this book: Plan ahead. Whether the terminally ill person is in the home or hospital, if advance planning has been done and dialogue has been held, these issues should have been discussed. If the patient has a funeral home and burial place preference, then obviously that should be honored, and that establishment may be consulted early. If hospice is involved, they will help with after-death issues. Hospital staffs will also take care of many of the post-death issues. If no funeral home is designated by the patient or family, hospitals or hospices will have a default resource. With a little foresight and discussion, after-death issues can be very manageable and need not be a source of anxiety.

On a practical note, one does not need to be concerned about the immediate post-death care of the body. Nothing alarming will happen in the first few hours. The body will simply cool and lose color. Rush and panic are not required. Usually a phone call is all that is needed to set the after-death care in motion.

Notes

10

End-of-Life Care
in the Nursing Home

Lance writes . . .

Nursing home care is appropriate for a wide variety of health problems. Many nursing home residents will eventually return to their homes after a period of rehabilitation or convalescence. However, the discussion of end-of-life care is not complete without consideration of terminal illness in the nursing home environment.

For better or worse, many people in our society spend their final days of life in a nursing home. Some people are admitted to nursing homes with progressive diseases such as dementia or terminal cancer, and there is no expectation they will ever go home again. Eventually they will die in the nursing home. Other individuals may go into a nursing home with the hope that diseases or problems will improve with therapy and attention, but instead the patients get worse quickly and ultimately enter the dying process. In any case, it is important that we try to arrange for good end-of-life care, just as we would in any other setting.

I believe the five principles of *The Active Management of Dying* should be our guide in the nursing home. They are broad enough to be of use in almost any setting where a person might experience stages of dying. Please note that I tend to use the terms *patient, resident,* and *client* interchangeably when referring to a person receiving care in the nursing home.

Let's review the principles of *The Active Management of Dying:*

1. Accept the reality of the situation.

2. Identify the decision-makers.

3. Discuss the ultimate goals of care.

4. Create an end-of-life care plan.

5. Implement the care plan you created.

Nursing Home Resources

Let us now consider the resources available in the nursing home environment. Granted, nursing homes vary tremendously in every conceivable category, from available space to quality of food to the ratio of staff to residents. However, I will try to make useful generalizations for your basic understanding.

Social Workers. Most nursing homes have a full- or part-time social worker. Sometimes a *nurse coordinator* may be doing the same job. This person serves a vital role. His or her duties usually will include coordinating patient and family concerns, participating in treatment/care planning, helping with evaluation of behavioral/psychiatric abnormalities, and assisting with discharge planning. Often the social worker has the primary responsibility for discussing end-of-life issues with patients and families. For example, the social worker might present a newly admitted patient and family with a packet of information, including living wills and the forms to designate a health care power of attorney, and provide assistance understanding them. The social worker will probably seek to identify a family spokesperson or health care power of attorney. Certainly, these basic components of end-of-life care should be universal. It is hoped, as we have said many times before, that these discussions and documentations would be initiated long before a crisis or advanced stage of dying occur.

Nurses. Obviously, there will be nurses in a nursing home. They will vary in terms of experience and training, but they are the glue that holds the facility together. They administer medications, triage and treat medical issues in conjunction with the doctors, and participate in care planning with the whole team. Often the nurse will also do many of the jobs of the social worker and may offer guidance on end-of-life documents.

It is fair to say the nurses usually will be highly knowledgeable about the details of patients' medical care, and the doctors will need the nurses' insights to properly evaluate patients. The relationships formed between patients, nurses, and the families during long nursing home stays can become very deep. Good relationships among these three parties are crucial to ensuring optimal nursing home care, and this is especially true for end-of-life care. Poor relationships with poor communication will result in confusion and sluggish decision-making that may create additional chaos for the dying person.

Aides/Technicians. Utmost respect must be given to these hands-on workers who attend to the daily needs of some of society's most frail and vulnerable members. The aide or technician serves as the body and mind that the patient no longer has. If the patients can no longer move themselves around, feed themselves, dress themselves, use the toilet, clean themselves, or even turn over in bed, someone will be responsible for getting that done. It is difficult and underpaid work, but without it many people would have a hellish existence during an already difficult time. I will say without hesitation that I have been deeply moved and humbled by these people who demonstrate such honest compassion on a daily basis. I honestly do not know how they muster the strength for it each day, but I'm profoundly grateful that they do.

Rehabilitation Services. Nursing homes always have some availability of physical therapy, as well as speech, occupational, and recreational therapy. Some facilities have full- or part-time professional staff to provide this, while others use visiting consultants for individual patients who may benefit.

Several beneficial goals may be accomplished through the use of such services. Some patients recover strength and function, enabling them to go home. For others, they maintain the ability to care for themselves longer. For the very ill, the bed-bound, or the severely demented, rehabilitative services may help to slow the development of bedsores or pneumonias. The therapists, through their interactions with the client, may identify changes in the pain level or other changes in status that would otherwise go unnoticed. Often the simple act of movement that the therapist facilitates may be a major source of pain relief for a bed-bound or wheelchair-bound patient.

Medical Directors. Although nursing homes rarely have a full time physician at the facility, a nursing home must have a physician named as the *medical director*. This doctor has administrative duties as well as clinical responsibilities. The medical director will seek to keep the facility in compliance with national guidelines. He or she will work to develop medical policies for the whole facility. Some patients in the nursing home will have private physicians who organize their care and prescribe medications and treatments. For those who do not have a private attending physician, the medical director will serve that role or find another physician to do so. The medical director will be aware of end-of-life issues and may facilitate various parts of the planning.

I should caution you that the medical director may not know all the details of a particular patient's case, especially if another doctor is the primary physician. I have heard families become very concerned when the medical director cannot immediately answer detailed questions about their loved one's condition, even when that patient has another doctor making the ultimate care decisions. Usually the medical director will consult the nurse, the medical record, and the primary doctor if a family has a question he or she cannot answer.

Primary Physicians. Some clients have their own physicians who will follow them in the nursing home. We have already discussed the tremendous value of having a primary doctor who knows the patient well. The primary doctor will order medications and treatments, examine the patient at regular intervals, and make decisions about the appropriate type of environment: Should the patient be in a hospital, nursing home, residential home, or the patient's actual home? Ideally, the primary doctor would be proactively involved in any end-of-life planning and will have the trust and respect of the patient and family.

Nutrition Services. Another valuable, yet often overlooked, service in the nursing home is the food. I hope the reader does not laugh and think I am saying that nursing home food is universally gourmet cuisine. Trust me, I have eaten enough institutional food to know better. However, nursing homes do provide good and consistent nutrition to those who otherwise might not receive it.

A very interesting phenomenon occurs somewhat commonly in

nursing homes. Many of the chronic diseases with a significant nutritional component, such as diabetes, high blood pressure, and heart disease, actually improve or even disappear in the nursing home. It is really quite simple—the clients are prescribed special diets for their conditions, such as low salt, low sugar, low fat, and so forth, and that's what they get. At home they may have had difficulty following their diets, and the disease stayed out of control, requiring multiple medications and high doses. Also, remember that as people approach death they tend to eat less and less, which alone reduces high blood sugar and high blood pressure. It is indeed ironic that nursing home life and the dying process can actually treat, even cure, some of our most common and devastating diseases. So, you should not be too surprised if you notice that the doctor takes away some patients' long-term medications as they near the end of life.

Strategies for Optimizing Nursing Home Care

I made a point of introducing you to some of the key figures in the nursing home setting for a very specific reason. The more you understand the importance of each staff member, the more likely you are to develop a good relationship with those individuals. Thus a team spirit may flourish. Remember that our ultimate goal is to improve end-of-life care for the dying person. A cooperative team is crucial and nowhere more so than the nursing home.

The patient and/or family must understand the daily challenges and heartaches that the nursing home staff faces on a daily basis. They constantly deal with disease, decay, and death. They clean the feces, urine, and blood for people to whom they are not even related. They wrestle with difficult governmental regulations. They often take the brunt of pain, frustration, and fear from patients and families despite their best efforts to alleviate those things. Even at their best they are often overwhelmed with day-to-day realities. It has been my experience that despite all these hurdles, nursing home staffs do a miraculous job of caring for their clients.

The best thing you can do if your loved one is in a nursing home, to ensure that they will receive excellent attention, is to develop a rapport with the staff. I am not saying the staff would neglect a patient otherwise. I am saying that the staff is made up of human beings. If they know the family well and feel comfortable with them, and vice versa, the conversations will be easier and more honest. The staff will naturally want to spend some extra time with the client and family.

Let's briefly discuss the ugly reality of abuse and neglect of clients in nursing homes. It happens. It is rare. It is wrong. It is criminal. However, it is easy to be confused by certain things in the nursing home. There are some patients who are not in control of themselves due to brain disease and must be physically restrained for the safety of all. Others must have wound care that can cause discomfort. Other patients are demented and may react to normal care as if they are being abused.

If you have a family member in a nursing home and you have concerns about his or her care or treatment, address it immediately, but respectfully, to the senior person on the staff. The odds are there is a reasonable explanation for the activity in question. Keep an open mind because the staff may be dealing with difficulties that you have not encountered before. I have seen the staff being abused much more often than I have seen patients being abused. Of course if the explanation or behavior is or becomes unacceptable, or if there is blatant abuse or neglect, the patient's situation should be addressed immediately with the nursing home and also with proper authorities such as the Department of Health and the police.

Here is a common scenario: A severely demented patient is admitted to the nursing home, and the family comes to visit occasionally.

The patient becomes violent during bathing and tries to strike the staff. The staff uses approved methods to humanely restrain the patient's arms while sponge bathing is done. A family member comes to visit and is unprepared for this sight. He walks in during sponge bathing and sees his mother "tied down." He immediately flies into a rage and begins accusing the staff of abusing his mother. The reality was that the patient was getting a necessary bath and was not harmed, but the staff is burdened with defending themselves from the accusations. This is an extreme example, but I have seen it occur more than once. It would have been much better if the son were simply to ask why the restraints were being used. If he were aware of some of the reasons why such actions are taken, then the scene would be less traumatic for all.

An unfortunate reality of human decline is the progressive loss of bodily control that many people experience. For most of our lives after early childhood, we move on our own, attend to our own toileting and hygiene, feed ourselves, and dress ourselves. Once we lose that capacity due to advanced disease or senility, we essentially regress back to an infantile state. Think about how much care an infant needs. Imagine an infant in the body of an adult. The adult body is heavier and there is more surface area to clean. Sometimes infants soil their diapers and the diaper is often not changed right away. The bottom line is that when a person is unable to take care of their daily needs, it takes an incredible amount of work to do it for them. Sometimes families of patients in nursing homes believe that their family member who is in such a situation will stay immaculately cared for at all times because they are in a nursing home level of care. It is important to temper those expectations. Even in the best nursing homes, patients may wait a bit for cleanings and turnings. Helping the staff with such duties will be very much appreciated. Good care should be expected, but perfect care is impossible. Optimal care is a team effort.

Specific End-of-Life Issues

If it seems that I have been discussing generalities about nursing home care, rather than specifics about end-of-life care in the nursing home, it's because the two concepts are clearly related. End-of-life care in the nursing home is really about the same as other forms of care, except with different goals. Ideally when a nursing home patient enters a comfort or palliative care model they will simply have a shift in their medications, reducing disease-altering medications and increasing comfort medications. The proper documentation will be in place so the nursing home staff will not feel compelled to initiate extreme measures to forestall death late in the process.

Hospice in the Nursing Home

Hospice services can be used in the nursing home just like they can at a private residence. Hospice benefits can be used to supplement the nursing care already provided in the nursing home and generally only require a physician's certification that the life expectancy is six months or less. Nursing homes are usually able to accommodate all medications and comfort measures requested by the attending physician, but with hospice on board, the patient and family may get even more attention.

Hospice houses are more common in densely populated urban areas than in more rural areas. A hospice house is staffed by hospice nurses and workers and is specifically designed to care for the needs of those who are dying. For patients and families for whom death at their own home is not an option, a hospice house may be viewed as a very good alternative. I would recommend them to anyone searching for a place to receive end-of-life care.

Documentation

If a patient is to receive end-of-life care in a nursing home or hospice, the documentation is just as important as it is in the home or hospital. Efforts should be made to obtain and sign the living will, health care power of attorney, and bedside EMS Do Not Resuscitate forms. I feel strongly that the attending physician should write specific orders in the chart outlining the scope of treatment and conditions for transport to the hospital. Ideally, if the end-of-life plan is solid, the patient will not be transported to the hospital, and treatment of specific problems (pneumonia, for example) would be minimized.

The Bottom Line

Nursing homes can be very challenging environments, and the staffs are usually excellent people trying to do compassionate work. They are human and therefore not perfect. Optimal nursing home care in general, and especially end-of-life care, will be improved when all parties work together to support the dying person. Expectations need to be realistic, and families who assist with the care of their loved ones will enhance the overall care tremendously. Frequent, honest, and respectful communication and documentation are crucial to the whole process.

Bert writes...

We can all readily understand why the move to a nursing home is very hard for many people. It usually means the dissolution of one's familiar home. That is a great loss, like a little death.

The move often requires leaving cherished neighbors and places behind. The furniture, bric-a-brac, pictures, and books that one has to give away or sell are all loaded with tons of unique memories and special meaning. That's a lot of loss heaped on top of the loss of physical abilities that has made the move to the nursing home necessary.

All the losses involved in moving to the nursing home have to be acknowledged so the person can grieve them. Even when it appears the new environment is going to be better in every way, the loss of things in the old environment is significant and shouldn't be glossed over. This can be a family conversation when a family is involved, because everyone's life is changing. Recognize that a person's life story is embedded in the things that furnish his or her home. Talking about all these things in detail, listening to the stories they evoke, and feeling the emotions connected with them in empathy with the aging parent who must now let them go, can help heal the wounds of loss.

Yet it's not all loss and grieving and letting go, important as that is. The conversation can also move to things the resident can realistically look forward to. Lance has alluded to real advantages in nursing home living, when health and independence can actually be improved and where one need not always be alone.

The important point is to talk about these things, openly and in detail, so that both letting go and hoping for the best can make this major transition a graceful one.

A Note to Caregivers

Lance spoke about the conditions for optimal nursing home care. He has learned that the main feature of optimal care is genuine collaboration among all the parties involved. Collaboration, he said, requires realistic expectations and honest, respectful communication between each family member and the patient.

The sacred work of tending the needs of persons at the end of life makes the nursing home no place for turf wars. Everyone there brings valuable skills, perspectives, and resources to the common task. When real collaboration is the rule—and I have seen this happen beautifully—the patient's loss of familiar things at home can be compensated by recreating another home where everyone feels support and safety and belonging.

Only when staff members feel support, safety, and belonging is it likely that the patients will have that experience.

What strategies improve collaboration? Let me suggest four that seem especially important for the professional caregiver:

1. Take up your professional authority and use it with flexibility. Your role is needed both in decision-making and in carrying out the functions of the place, and you should exercise your role with confidence. But there is usually more than one way to get a task done. Confident people can bend. When there are frustrations, deal with them quickly and honestly.

2. Keep focused on the patient. When the momentum of work is focused on the patient and family needs, and not on rigid role definitions (turf) or issues of personal status or ego, teamwork is fluid and purposeful. The real business at hand is to care for the patient.

3. Recognize your limits and boundaries, as well as your areas of strength. This makes it natural to value team members' contributions. Who would dare trust only his or her own head when making important health care decisions for someone else?

4. Tempering confidence with humility serves the patient best and also decreases unnecessary stress for you.

Stay emotionally and spiritually healthy. Needy, depleted people inevitably use their professional roles to get their own needs met, which means they are not free to serve the needs of the patient or family. Self-care and tending not only ensure your happiness; self-care and tending are an ethical mandate.

The Hospice Perspective

I want to amplify Lance's reference to hospice care. More information is given about hospice in Appendix A, including what hospices are and what they do. Here, we simply endorse the hospice perspective or philosophy on end-of-life care. It is valid for nursing homes too.

The genius of hospice is that it defines spiritual, emotional, and social (relationship) suffering and care as being equally important as physical suffering and care. Make no mistake—physical pain is never disregarded and every effort is made to ease pain. But the whole person is always kept in view, and that makes all the difference.

Notes

11

End-of-Life Care Issues
in the Intensive Care Unit

Lance writes . . .

Although I am not a specialist in intensive care medicine, I have taken care of quite a few patients there. I am confident my colleagues in the intensive care unit (ICU) will support what I say here. As we have said, the general principles of *The Active Management of Dying* can apply to any setting, including the ICU. Keep them in mind as we go through some of the particular issues.

The Active Management of Dying

1. Accept the reality of the situation.

2. Identify the decision-makers.

3. Discuss the ultimate goals of care.

4. Create an end-of-life care plan.

5. Implement the care plan you created.

The ICU is a life-support center. Most patients in an ICU are so sick, injured, or burned that they literally depend on tubes and machines for their minute-to-minute survival. Breathing tubes and ventilators may supply each breath, and may be delivering highly concentrated oxygen. Their blood pressure, pulse rate, cardiac function, kidney function, blood chemistries, blood volumes, and other vital processes may be so out of control that only continuous infusions (drips) of powerful medications prevent death. Their entire fluid and nutrition intake may be controlled through lines and tubes, as they are 'not capable of dealing with their own requirements for these. They may be undergoing intensive dialysis if their kidneys have failed. They may be experiencing massive accumulations of fluid that require drainage or diuresis. In other words, machines, medications, and other people are taking the place of the person's own vital functions...which is, of course, "life support."

If you (layperson or professional) have a loved one or a patient in ICU, it is important that you keep in mind the goals of care. We will now look at different types of patients who receive ICU care, and the reasons why such intensive and invasive treatment is considered appropriate. These are generalizations, but, as always, we are trying to help you think through the main concepts.

The easiest cases involve patients with a single organ system problem, or who may be post-operative from an uncomplicated surgery, who were in reasonably good health previously, who will recover smoothly and transition soon to a lower intensity of care. Obviously, for patients such as these, one would not discuss or plan for end-of-life care, other than having one's advance directives already squared away (which we all should do when we are healthy).

Other patients are more complicated. They may have several diseases or injuries. It may be unclear as to why they are in such dangerous states of health, so a diagnosis and prognosis are not yet feasible. They may have a reasonable chance to "pull through" and recover, but the outcome is far from certain. In these patients, medical futility has not been reached, and we would all agree that intensive care is appropriate as we endeavor to bring the person back to an acceptable degree of health and quality of life. These people may go either way, however. Many will deteriorate and die despite every intervention, while others may surprise everyone with their resiliency and will to live, showing great recovery despite the odds.

In addition to having advance directives in place, I strongly advise the family and the medical team to begin some early "what if" discussions for patients who are in questionable status. "What if things get worse instead of better?" "What if she ends up completely dependent on these machines and medications with no hope of recovery?" Basically, in these people we hope for the best (and do everything to increase the odds), but we should also prepare for the worst. Again, if we live in denial of unpleasant possibilities, we may fail to provide optimal end-of-life planning and care if things do not go as we hope.

Then there is the group who has clearly reached medical futility. Perhaps they entered the ICU with a reasonable chance of recovery, but their bodies simply could not overcome whatever insult put them there, or new complications (infections, other diseases) arise and change the course significantly. Perhaps they entered the ICU with a poor chance of recovery, but the doctor or the family felt compelled to try all measures before giving up, and then those measures failed. Sometimes patients with no chance of recovery are kept alive for some period of time in the ICU. This may be done in order to give the family time to assemble and come to terms with the impending death. Other times it gives the ICU physician or the primary care physician a chance to go over the whole record and be sure that all is in order (the patient may have been admitted by another doctor). Some patients are kept mechanically alive after brain death so their organs can be taken for transplant to another person (we will discuss that a bit later). Whatever the case, these patients will eventually be identified and decisions will have to be made about withdrawing these intense interventions (we will discuss that too).

ICU Pitfalls

It is also important for you to understand that patients who are sick enough to require ICU care are by definition very fragile, and that you be aware of some of the complications that may arise despite the best efforts of the ICU team. Keeping a human being alive by artificial life support comes with much risk, and the therapies themselves may further damage the person, even while saving them from imminent death.

Infections. Since the sickest patients go to the ICU, the worst infections and a high concentration of infected people will be found there. Many of the organisms (germs) that infect ICU patients are resistant to many of our best antibiotics (a tremendous problem facing us all) and the diseases they cause are devastating to anyone, especially someone who is already critically ill. Additionally, ICU patients are usually bed-bound, which dramatically increases the likelihood of lung, skin, and urinary tract (bladder and kidney) infections that the person who moves around independently would not suffer.

Ventilator dependence. While breathing tubes and ventilators may save lives in those who cannot breathe for themselves, many intubated patients are too sick and weak to ever come back off the machine and live. Patients with end-stage lung and heart disease are prime examples. Sometimes, during the emergent act of placing a breathing tube to save a life (intubating), damage to the airway and lungs will inadvertently occur and further complicate the ability of the patient to recover. Other times, a patient may have already suffered irreversible brain damage due to lack of oxygen prior to the artificial respiration, and this will not be realized for some time.

Oxygen toxicity. We all need oxygen to survive, and patients with lung disease may need high concentrations of it to get enough across the lung tissue and into circulation. Ironically, though, oxygen itself is toxic in high doses. An apple turns brown after it's exposed to atmospheric oxygen. Lung tissues suffer similar damage from long-term, high-dose oxygen exposure, even though it may be necessary for immediate survival. This may complicate recovery from the original lung problem.

Drug reactions and allergies. Any drug can cause adverse affects and dangerous allergic reactions. Even medications that a person is accustomed to can occasionally cause a surprise reaction. Imagine a critically ill person requiring high doses of multiple powerful medications just to stay alive. It is not hard to see that the risk of problems caused by the lifesaving medications increases rapidly. Of course we do not use a medicine unless the benefit is felt to outweigh the risks. But, in a critically ill person, the alternative of not using the medication is often death, making the stakes very high.

Blood clots. A very dangerous and common problem found in bedbound patients, cancer patients, and patients with blood diseases is that of blood clot formation in the deep veins (deep vein thrombosis or DVT), which may break loose and cause life-threatening blockages in the circulation of the heart (heart attack), lungs (pulmonary embolism), or brain (stroke). ICU patients are at particular risk of DVT formation. There are mechanical and medical methods to reduce this risk, but they are not perfect.

Bed sores. The bed-bound ICU patient is also at high risk of developing serious bed sores that are then at risk for developing infections from those tough, resistant germs that plague the ICU. Despite our best efforts, when patients cannot move on their own, they are probably going to develop skin breakdown over pressure areas. These sores are often painful, unpleasant, and very slow to heal, even if the person leaves the ICU.

Multi-organ system failure. This clinical entity is not perfectly understood, but may be the final blow that takes the life of a critically ill person. The human body is a delicately balanced system of organs working together to sustain life. If an organ is severely damaged or diseased, a cascade of events may be triggered that eventually affects other organ systems, and the body seems to actually turn on itself. This cascade may spread like wildfire through the body and cause death despite very aggressive efforts to stop it.

ICU Psychosis. Just being in the ICU is enough to literally drive some people insane, to the point that they may rip out the very lines and tubes that are keeping them alive. Add the fact that the patients are already sick and drugged, and you have a situation where patients may suddenly and unexpectedly cause themselves unintentional harm. All patients are monitored closely to reduce the likelihood of damaging themselves, but their status can change quickly and it only takes a few seconds to get out of control.

Iatrogenic injury. This refers to inadvertent injury caused to the patient by the health care professional while attempting to properly treat the patient. Despite precautions and skill, these unfortunate events do occur from time to time. Every procedure and every medication we use in health care carries some degree of risk. We try not to use any intervention unless the potential benefits outweigh the risk. Unless it is an emergency and/or the patient does not have capacity and no one is available to speak for him or her, we do get informed consent before any invasive procedure and discuss the risks and benefits.

Now, let us imagine a critically ill or injured patient in the ICU. Just to resuscitate and stabilize the patient from the initial insult (in other words the flurry of activity required to save his life), he may have had several major invasive, and sometimes painful, procedures in an emergent fashion. Each day he may require new procedures, which also may be emergent, to diagnose and treat his problems and subsequent complications. Since each ICU patient usually will have several procedures and medications, and each procedure and medication has some risk associated even under the best of circumstances, and each ICU has several patients, it is inevitable that iatrogenic injury may sometimes occur.

The reality is that as we do our best to save lives, we will occasionally do some harm to a small number of individuals. It is a price we pay. The obvious question, "Is iatrogenic injury a sign of malpractice?" is usually answered no. It is usually an unfortunate consequence of a very complicated and dramatic form of medical care. The important thing is that the doctor be straightforward with the patient and family if an iatrogenic injury occurs, explaining what happened and what can be done about it.

Strategies for Optimizing ICU End-of-Life Care

In the nursing home chapter, we talked about team building and good communication as important strategies for giving the dying person the best possible care (as it would be valuable in any situation). We have spoken at length about the value of an identified surrogate for the incapacitated patient. Given the pace and complexity of ICU care, you already realize that these same strategies are absolutely vital for any ICU patient whether the patient is actively recovering or *actively dying.*

So what role does the ICU actually play in end-of-life care? Hopefully, very little. For patients with incurable, medically futile problems, our goal is to do the groundwork far ahead of time that will avoid admission to the ICU. Remember, our goal for end-of-life care in terminally ill people who have reached medical futility is to keep them in comfortable, peaceful environments. In most cases, the ICU is quite the opposite of our goal.

But many people do die in the ICU, and often we know it will happen. Some of them die suddenly via cardiopulmonary arrest (a "code"), even when they may have been relatively stable immediately prior. For others, it is more complicated. I am referring to those people who received ICU care in an attempt to bring them back to a sustainable degree of health, but who simply will not make it. This results in a complicated end-of-life situation. We now have a person on life support whose time to die has clearly arrived, but who physically cannot die unless we take specific actions to allow it.

Withdrawal of Support

Let us imagine an elderly patient with multiple medical problems, including advanced lung disease (which would probably take his life soon anyway), who was admitted to the ICU on a ventilator after his own breathing failed. Let us say he does have advance directives in place and his daughter serves as his health care power of attorney. Imagine that although at first he had some slim hope of recovery from this particular crisis, his case gets more complicated over a few days. He develops a pneumonia caused by resistant bacteria. The infection spreads to his blood and causes sepsis, shock, and multi-organ system failure. No interventions improve the situation. In essence, he is actively dying, and is only "alive" because the machines force his lungs to keep expanding and the medications force his blood circulation to continue at some minimal level. His advance directives and his daughter's memory of his spoken wishes clearly indicate he would not want to be kept alive like this. His doctors believe medical futility has been reached. All are in agreement that nothing else should be done, and all are aware that death is imminent once the interventions are stopped.

This is a very common scenario, and although it looks bleak, there are a few bright spots. There are advance directives and a surrogate. Understanding and communication among the various team members is evident. Acceptance has been gained. Yet, there is still the uncomfortable work of actually withdrawing support. This means purposefully taking out breathing tubes and turning off ventilators, stopping medications and fluids, and halting any further life-supporting measures. In other words, the team will very dramatically and clearly act to let that person die. We will hope that good comfort measures would be initiated simultaneously. Perhaps the person would be moved to the regular hospital floor if the dying occurred slowly, or perhaps he or she might die there in the ICU.

In any event, the drama of the dying process will be distilled and concentrated. However, the principles and advice of *The Active Management of Dying* remain constant and applicable here as well. Conversely, you can also envision scenes in which things are less well-organized. Perhaps there is no advance directive or no surrogate, or the surrogate does not feel she knows the patient's wishes. Imagine how chaotic and guilt-ridden the situation could quickly become. Again, good planning will clearly serve to reduce the angst of even the worst situations.

Other Ethical Issues in the ICU

Withdrawal of support is the subject of tremendous consideration. ICU care in general brings to mind two other important ethical issues that deserve discussion. The first is organ donation. Many organ donors will suffer brain death, and then their bodies will be sustained mechanically in the ICU until the donated organs can be surgically given to a viable (living) recipient. The advance directives and surrogates usually will be crucial to the decision-making process involved in organ donation.

The second is the concept of stewardship. By this I mean the responsible use of limited resources. ICU care requires vast amounts of resources of many types, and decisions made about the type of care given can have tremendous impacts on the resources used.

Of course these issues are important in many other settings but the ICU distills them and dramatically demonstrates their relevance. They will receive a more in depth discussion later in the book.

The Bottom Line

ICU physicians and surgeons are among the most highly skilled and trained professionals you will find anywhere. They deal with problems of an incredible magnitude and frequently save lives that would otherwise have been lost. But they are still imperfect human beings treating other imperfect human beings, and they will lose many patients despite heroic attempts. ICU care comes at a tremendous cost, and good outcomes are not guaranteed. I do not say this to paint a depressing picture, rather to help you stay out of the "denial trap." If the situation requires, I want you to be ready to move quickly and confidently into end-of-life planning. I have seen many cases of family members and inexperienced physicians-in-training who were stunned by the speed and complexity of cases in the ICU. They spent a lot of valuable time trying to understand medical details when time was of the essence and big-picture decisions were crucial. I am trying to help you avoid that wasted time and powerlessness by arming you with a basic understanding long before a crisis.

Notes

12

End-of-Life Care Issues
in the Emergency Department

Lance writes . . .

I am a family physician by training but have worked primarily as an emergency physician for the last four years. I have staffed emergency departments (EDs) of all sizes: small rural communities, level-one trauma centers, indigent county hospitals, and the sands of Iraq. This broad medical and social perspective has been invaluable and helps me to keep my perspective on end-of-life issues in the ED.

The ED is usually the worst place for a dying patient. End-of-life planning should specifically aim to keep people out of ED care. Our goal is to keep the dying person comfortable, and the ED is one of the most uncomfortable places one can be. Unfortunately, life is uncertain, and many hospice and comfort-care patients do end up there. I will describe the role and staff of the ED for your understanding, and then give you some strategies for optimizing care there, should it become necessary.

The ED is designed to stabilize and treat patients with emergent, often obscure problems. The primary job is to save life, limb, and sight. It is a chaotic world that takes all comers at all hours. It is impossible to predict what problems will be encountered on any given day because there are no appointments and no control over when patients will arrive. Sometimes it's so busy that patients line the halls on gurneys, and other times hours may go by without a patient. Emergency physicians and nurses see that their purpose is to prevent anyone from dying on their shifts. They want to make rapid decisions about treatment and where the patient will go next, and then move on to the next patient. Those patients with obvious life-threatening issues will be triaged to the front of the line while others may wait hours to be seen. Emergency physicians cannot afford the time to form long-term relationships with patients. During busy times they must continually move from patient to patient, treating immediate problems and determining who goes into the hospital and who goes home. Spending too much time with any one patient means that another may not get seen in a timely fashion, and that could have fatal results. ED physicians must also deal with the constant risk of lawsuits. Because they do not have the time to form relationships with patients and because of the severe problems they manage, ED physicians often take the brunt of the legal consequences of bad medical outcomes. Therefore, they tend to do extensive tests and admit patients to the hospital, rather than develop outpatient treatment strategies.

Let us now imagine a typical end-of-life case in the ED. An elderly man with advanced colon cancer and several other medical problems is living at home with family. His cancer was recently deemed incurable, and even attempts to provide palliative radiation are failing—the tumors are growing despite attempts to slow them. During his last hospitalization, a Do Not Resuscitate order was placed on the hospital chart and hospice was discussed, but no specific end-of-life plans were made. Recently, he stopped eating, has become very weak, and no longer talks. Although his family has a general sense that there is no further benefit to medical intervention, they panic and bring him to the ED at 6:30 PM during a very busy rush. The emergency physician has a quick conversation with the family, and they do not assert any real preferences for comfort care versus interventional care. The physician does a quick exam, orders some basics labs, and moves on to the next patient. When the labs come back, it is clear the man is dehydrated and malnourished. The emergency physician then calls the patient's regular doctor and arranges for admission, thinking the patient will get fluids and a feeding tube. The emergency physician is aware that the patient is under DNR orders, but knows that this is not a resuscitation issue. He feels that his job is done. The patient stays in the hospital several days and a feeding tube is placed. Comfort measures are not well addressed as the feeding tube is the main focus. He is discharged home with another unclear plan.

This case represents the common (and understandable) style of the ED. The physician does an adequate job with the patient and certainly maintains the overall patient flow, which he must do. The family was probably overwhelmed by the chaos of the ED and did not understand how to assert any wishes. The physician was forced to move onto the next patient before the family had a chance to formulate any questions. Is this bad medicine? No, it is not. The ED physician probably sees end-of-life issues as the responsibility of the primary physician or oncologist, and there are many who would agree with that. We cannot fault him for his management, and if he had failed to move on to a critically ill child, then he would have been an incompetent physician indeed. Does this case demonstrate an optimal level of care? Certainly not. There are several points where the decisions and communication could have been improved on the part of both the family and the doctor, even in a very busy ED. Of course, with good foresight and planning, we could have prevented the patient from ever being at the mercy of ED chaos in the first place.

Optimizing End-of-Life Care in the ED

Once again, I will ask you to reflect on the principles of *The Active Management of Dying* as we examine this particular environment. Once again, I will name teamwork and honest, assertive communication as the cornerstones of optimal end-of-life care in the ED.

The ED can be a poor place to do end-of-life planning and care, but there is some potential for productive dialogue and planning. When the ED is very busy, we will obviously have limited involvement with any individual patient, but sometimes the ED is quiet and there are very few patients. During these periods, the emergency physician may have the opportunity to explore options for hospice and comfort measures with the family and help to get the dying person home rather than admitted to the hospital. When the patient and family arrive at the ED with an understanding of the dying process, the constraints of emergency care, and a clear idea of the overall plan for the patient, they will find the interaction to be much more productive and empowering.

Let us now take the same patient as above, put him back into the busy ED, but illustrate some differences in the course. You remember that he had end-stage colon cancer and was receiving ineffective palliative radiation. He had recently stopped taking fluid and nutrition. He had a hospital DNR order on record but the details of his care plan were not set. Hospice had not yet been consulted. So let's imagine that his family becomes concerned about his recent deterioration. Although they sense that he is moving into the dying process, and they have some knowledge on the subject thanks to reading and discussion, they remain unsure about what to do and call EMS. Upon arrival to the emergency department, they realize it is very busy. While waiting for the doctor, they take a moment to organize their information about the patient and his medications. They list their questions and wishes for the doctor and agree to let one family member be the spokesperson. When the doctor arrives at the bedside the spokesperson lets the doctor know the family is aware the patient is dying, but they want an idea of how imminent the death is and need some time to prepare for it. The doctor examines the hospital records, does an examination and some basic tests on the patient, and determines that the patient is indeed dying. He does not expect death is imminent. The team is working together well, but the ED is full. The emergency physician then recommends that the patient be admitted for a short while to give the primary physician or oncologist a chance to coordinate care and get hospice involved. He also documents the DNR status and family's desire to move toward comfort measures only. The family is relieved. The primary physician accepts the admission and is grateful that the ED physician has already done ground work that prevents a complicated hospital stay full of inappropriate expectations. After one day the patient goes home under hospice care. The hospital social worker provides the family with advance directive documents and an Out-of-Hospital DNR order. The family commits to keeping the patient comfortable at home for his remaining time. He dies peacefully one week later, with his family and a hospice worker in attendance.

Even better results can be seen when the ED is slow and all parties work well toward the common goal of comfort care. Imagine the above patient arrives at the ED at 11:00 PM, after the daily rush is over. His family is organized as above, and now the emergency physician takes a little more time with this patient because there are no compelling distractions. He reviews the record and discusses the case with the patient's oncologist who confirms that medical futility has been reached and supports a move toward definite comfort care. The emergency physician then offers to make an immediate hospice referral and begin comfort medications in the ED. The nurses agree to observe the patient in the ED while the family makes arrangements with hospice and the hospital social worker over the next two hours. The patient then goes home comfortably three hours after arriving in the ED. The family is well pleased, and the doctor has done excellent work. The patient dies a few days later in his own bed. There are no regrets.

If you think I am over-idealizing the role of the ED physician or the capacity of the family to affect change, I can tell you confidently that I am not. I practice end-of-life care in the ED several times per week in exactly that fashion, and know of colleagues who do the same. It never fails to leave me with a sense of satisfaction to know that the patient, family, staff, and I came together quickly to form a team and a plan. I routinely follow-up with these families and find they were invariably pleased with the care we provided. I strongly recommend that terminally ill patients and their families avoid the ED whenever possible. However, if they must go, I encourage them to be strong and clear in their plans. I implore my colleagues in emergency medicine to stay open to other options for their terminal patients, and to go the extra mile when time allows. More detailed suggestions are provided later in the book for the patient, family, and health professional in training.

Bert writes . . .

Emergency medicine has high dramatic value on TV, but in real life, as Lance points out, you don't want to go there if you can avoid it. When you have a thoughtful plan for the care of a loved one close to the end of life, a rushed trip to the ED usually won't have to happen. Still, it takes a lot of courage and stamina to resist calling the EMS when visible changes occur, even anticipated ones. I remember a young family doctor who once spent most of a Saturday evening at the home of a patient in hospice care. He had asked the family to call him rather than EMS if any disturbing change occurred, and they did. The doctor's reassurance kept the family from panic and he was able to hold them steady as they watched their loved one go through the last stages of dying. What could otherwise have been a futile and enervating experience in the ED became a calm and prayerful presence with the loved one. The family regained the composure and basic intentions that had originally led them the hospice way.

The role that physician played with the family on the verge of panic could be filled by a hospice worker, a pastor, a nurse, or a family member—whoever steps forward to remind the family of its basic commitments when the crisis occurs. Even then, sometimes the patient will be transported to the ED. I am glad Lance showed us how compassionate emergency staff, when not under a lot of pressure, can make the ED more conducive to the same careful planning for a peaceful death that may occur in other settings.

Notes

13

Special Considerations

Organ Donation

Lance writes . . .

I consider the subject of organ donation to be relevant to, but distinct from, the discussion of end-of-life care. The goal of providing optimal end-of-life care to an individual is an end in itself. Salvaging useable organs from the deceased to help the living is also an end in itself. However, there will be natural bridges between the two, and we will briefly explore some of those relationships.

I say again that *The Active Management of Dying* and well planned end-of-life care are best suited for those who have long-term progressive diseases, for which there is time to sort through the issues. Let's acknowledge that those same people are not usually good candidates to be organ donors because their organs were already in a poor state of health. The ideal organ donor is the tragic opposite. He or she is healthy and young, and died unexpectedly. Usually trauma, rather than long-term disease, would be the cause of death. Ironically, those people are usually the least likely to have done any end-of-life considerations.

However, neither of those generalizations is absolute. Some organs and tissues from people with long-term diseases, who go through a definable dying process, can be used to help others. It is up to the transplant specialists to decide on each case. Similarly, it should be noted that young people are asked about organ donation on most state driver's licenses, and can have more detailed wishes expressed and documented once they reach adulthood.

The decision to be an organ donor is obviously a very personal one, and the medical system shows great respect for such a decision. The time surrounding the dying process is the worst time to consider the sobering but important possibility of organ donation, as there are already so many decisions to make and emotions to experience. The best time to think about it is long before it becomes an issue. The legalities and processes of organ transplantation are highly specialized and beyond the scope of this book, but there are some important points you can consider.

When you are doing end-of-life planning, please discuss organ donation with those involved, and do not wait until the issue is at hand before getting it on the table. If possible it would be a very selfless gift to declare oneself an organ donor, and let it be known (both in spoken and written form). A good example would be to state, "If the transplant people feel someone else can use something of mine after I am gone, then I want them to have it." That gives the transplant agencies the best number of options.

I have known many families who had some confusion and concerns during the decision-making process as they considered approving organ donation on behalf of a deceased member. I have never known any who regretted it once they knew of the life that organ later saved. All of the families I have worked with whose deceased member donated an organ, later viewed the heroism of that act as the crowning positive event in the story of that person's life.

There are those who will refuse to be an organ donor and will not let their family members be organ donors either. Some cite religious reasons. Others say they simply cannot bear the thought of it. Others cannot verbalize a reason. Again, there is great respect for this decision, and no one in our society can or should be pressured into donating against his or her conscience.

There is one mindset that troubles me, and I have encountered it only rarely. I have met people who state that they would never allow themselves or their family members to be organ donors. However, at the same time, they do say they that would not only accept a donated organ if it would save their life or a family member's, but indeed would expect to have it. The basic problem here is obvious. There are many more people awaiting life-saving organ transplantation than there are suitable organs. Clearly, if there are those who would take without giving, then they will further deplete the pool of available organs. This seems fundamentally unfair. Therefore, I will ask that we all consider and discuss organ transplantation long before it becomes an issue. If someone would accept a transplanted organ in order to save his own life, then I think he must then try to offer the same chance to someone else. Blood donation is similar. There are many people whose disease state, even near the end of life, requires frequent transfusion of blood products to keep them alive, and whose families want that to continue. But that blood is part of a limited pool, so we must encourage the same families to donate blood when possible.

Bert writes . . .

When my father died of kidney failure in 1963, nothing could be done to prevent that kind of death. Today, with the same disease, he could be dialyzed and would probably receive a kidney transplant, and his life could be extended by many years at a high quality. Transplantation of non-renewable organs (such as kidney, liver, and heart) has developed into one of modern medicine's most successful ways of treating a wide variety of very serious diseases. The limiting factor, as Lance points out, is not the technology: it is the scarcity of organs available for transplant.

What keeps people from donating organs after death? For some, such as Orthodox Jews, religious beliefs about the sanctity of the body may prevent consent for the removal of organs after death. Very few religious groups hold beliefs that would exclude organ removal, however. Respect for the body does not exclude autopsy or organ removal for the purpose of donation, in the view of most religious traditions in the United States.

Others may be afraid that, in their eagerness to procure organs for transplantation, surgeons may hasten death or even remove organs before the patient has died. This fear is totally unfounded. The decision to remove a patient from life-sustaining treatment may be made only when there is no longer any benefit at all to the patient, and in consultation with the family. Then, the death of the donor must be determined by at least one doctor other than the organ recipient's physician, relying on current and available scientific tests. When the potential organ donor has been on life support, those tests usually determine whether or not "brain death" has occurred. When brain activity has completely and irreversibly stopped, the person is *dead*—even if machines are keeping the heart pumping artificially and if the chest appears to rise and fall as in breathing. Brain death means that the individual is really dead, with no possibility of recovery. Only after the physicians have declared the donor dead by their clinical judgment and by the laws of the state can the transplant procedure begin.

But for many of us, the reason we don't donate our organs for transplantation after death is that we simply never get around to it.

Even when I am motivated to "give back" or let a needy person use organs that I no longer have any use for, unless I take the initiative to consent to organ donation, it won't happen. If I do consent, or my surrogate consents for me, then it will happen and another life may be helped.

Stewardship

Lance writes . . .

I will be very honest here when I say that the decision to write this section came at the last minute before going to print. I did not want to alienate readers unfamiliar with the medical system, who might feel the discussion is too cold or asks too much of any individual or family. I decided to include this topic as I trust the reader to understand that this book is about helping—not just helping the individual, but all of us. It is no longer simply a professional talking with a client; it is about the sharing of ideas and looking at some very important fundamental issues. Please read the whole piece before reacting to it. I am not suggesting that one person martyr themselves for the good of all. On the contrary, good end-of-life care not only protects the individual from a chaotic and painful death, it protects valuable resources as well.

This book may have given you an appreciation for the complex nature of medical care. You see that keeping someone alive past a natural lifespan through interventions requires vast resources. Stewardship means taking care of what is placed under your control. Stewardship of resources implies conservation and judicious use. A child who remembers to turn out the lights when leaving a room delights parents who are proud of that stewardship of energy and family resources. Communities with outstanding recycling programs often win awards and grants to reward that form of stewardship. I don't think anyone feels good when we feel that we have squandered something precious, and I think we feel proud when we know we have preserved something for future generations. Stewardship can be viewed from a religious standpoint or a purely social standpoint, but either way it is vitally important.

I am reminded of a favorite song lyric, by a folk band called the Bo-Deans: "I'm takin' what I need, and I'm giving what I can...how much more can you ask of a man?" Being good stewards means we stay aware of what our actual needs are, and we avoid taking more than that.

You have probably noticed some recurring themes in this book. The development of antibiotic-resistant bacteria (germs) serves as a perfect focus. Antibiotics have been in existence for less than a century, but have become a cornerstone of modern medical practice. Early in their history, first-generation antibiotics cured previously fatal infections with miracle-like effectiveness. We probably went overboard and came to rely too much on these drugs, and used them far too often. In other words, we could have been better stewards of this powerful resource from the beginning. Less than a century later, we live in an age where that window of opportunity is closing rapidly. The toughest of those germs have survived the older antibiotics and have grown resistant to even our best and newest antibiotics. Now we are starting to see people succumb to infections that only a few years ago were easily cured by less powerful antibiotics. Each time we treat anyone with an antibiotic we risk contributing to the problem.

Does that mean we should stop using antibiotics? No, of course not. It means that we must become excellent stewards of this resource and use them only when there is a clear benefit. We must avoid using antibiotics for common colds (which do not respond to antibiotics anyway) in order to save them for a child with meningitis. We also must start to think about our current practice of treating infections in people who ought to be receiving comfort measures instead. I am *not* advocating that we withhold antibiotics just because someone is chronically ill. What I am saying is that we must be honest and courageous when dealing with people who are at the end of their natural lives. For those who are clearly entering the dying process, our compulsion should be to ease their suffering. We should not feel compelled to fight infections that are the natural result of decline.

Remember our case of Rev. Fisk? I recall how profoundly moved I was when his family made the decision to forego further treatments for his recurrent pneumonias. The decision was made when they realized the antibiotics were only delaying the inevitable, and their use in his case could put other people at risk. Once they understood the concept and saw it as an issue of stewardship, their decision was clear and easy.

The antibiotic resistance issue is just one example of how keeping a person alive artificially beyond medical benefit can waste vast amount of precious resources. Another example is ICU space. There are only so many beds available for intensive care and staff to run the units. If a person who cannot be improved from ICU care is kept on life support because the team is unable to accept the reality and move forward, then a valuable resource is consumed. Although most patients who can benefit from ICU care do receive it, delays due to lack of beds and staff can compromise that care. I doubt that any of us, if we were close to death and were not going to get better, would want to occupy an ICU bed that could benefit someone else.

Money should not be the driving force behind a medical decision. However, it is a tragedy when a lifetime of work is squandered. You must understand that many, many times entire estates have been exhausted because of the expense of caring for people who were years beyond their natural life and living in bed-bound misery. Let me be crystal clear once more. I am in no way suggesting that we put our most vulnerable people "out to pasture" so they can die and we can collect their inheritance. I am saying that when we exercise honesty about and acceptance of the end of our natural lives, we can exercise appropriate financial stewardship while keeping the individual comfortable and peaceful.

It is apparent that prolonged care in the ICU, hospital, or nursing home is extremely expensive. Whether the funding for that comes from the patient/family, from public pools like Medicare and Medicaid, or from private insurance, it does no one any good when we are spending that money without hope of benefit. In that vein, comfort care and hospice is incredibly more productive for both the dying patient and our society.

There is an ugly historical reality that is occasionally mentioned when one discusses end-of-life issues and resource stewardship. I have heard allusions to the horrors of Nazi Germany and other times when groups of people have tried to weed out members of society found "unworthy" of further existence, for the "benefit" of the larger society. There are also concerns over euthanasia. Bert discussed euthanasia earlier in the book. I will now say plainly and firmly, *The Active Management of Dying,* with good end-of-life care, is rooted firmly in the interests of the individual person. Any additional benefit to the larger society is a consideration, but only a secondary one. It has nothing to do with selecting out people and has everything to do with acknowledging the natural dying process we all may face. It is about keeping people empowered and dignified within the context of disease processes that have gone beyond human control. The discussion about stewardship of resources is not about withholding proper care from an individual for the profit of another, it is about respecting the finite nature of the resources we do have and using them only when they are of clear benefit. Regarding the controversial and awkward issue of euthanasia, we must remember that good end-of-life care serves to reduce the perceived need for euthanasia by giving the dying person other options.

With all that said...I should then clarify what I am suggesting. It is exactly what I have advocated throughout this book, fearless and honest communication in a proactive manner, before a crisis exists. I encourage you and your team (family and friends) to include in your end-of-life discussions some very frank questions about your legacy. Do you want to be remembered as an unselfish person who thought about the good of all? Do you want to preserve your estate for future generations of your family? Does your religious background consider stewardship as an important concept? What lessons do you want to teach the young ones? What strength and wisdom do you want to impart through your own demise? How do you feel about organ donation as a form of stewardship? I cannot possibly, nor would I want to, decide for you what role stewardship should or will play in your personal end-of-life planning. I am confident that your own reflections will guide you well. My goal is simply to get you to think about it deeply and discuss it with others.

Notes

14

Medications Commonly Used
in Terminal Care

Lance writes . . .

To help the reader gain a fuller understanding of the management of dying, it is helpful to know a bit about the medications commonly used to help the dying patient. This is not intended to be a pharmacology lecture. We will simply present an overview of the different classes of medications, examples of medications within that class, their actions, and some side effects. It is not possible to anticipate all the medications that might be used, but these are among the most likely to be encountered.

Narcotics

Also called opiates, these natural or synthetic derivatives of the poppy plant are primarily used for pain control. Different formulations are intended for various types of relief. Some are fast-acting and intended for short-term (acute) relief. Others are more slowly metabolized and intended for chronic (long-term) pain control. It is believed that opiates relieve pain primarily through disassociation and euphoria. In other words, they do not actually block the transmission of nerves that carry pain information to the brain, rather they put the patient in a state where they just do not care about the fact that pain exists. Since the body makes its own (endogenous) opiates (endorphins) that help us deal naturally with stress and pain, the exogenous (drug) opiates create the same effect to a much higher degree. Human beings who learn to control intense pain seem to do so by going into self-induced states that resemble a euphoric opioid condition.

Our society has much fear concerning the addictive potential of opiates, and perhaps with good reason. When healthy, thriving people becomes addicted to narcotics, their lives and the lives of those around them suffer. However, in the case of the dying patient, the priority shifts. The consequences are almost negligible if a dying person becomes addicted to narcotic pain relief once the dying process is clear.

I have been asked "What if a patient's dying process is prolonged and they develop tolerance to the narcotics, requiring increased doses for the same pain management effect?" To that I say, "Give them all they need. They are dying."

Opiates, in large doses, can suppress the patient's drive to breathe, which can cause or hasten death. Again, it is a different story when the patient has a chance to recover and live. In those patients, dosing is often more conservative. However, if the patient is very close to death and in severe pain, a dose of narcotic that is high enough to cause respiratory suppression may be justified if required to ease suffering. Comfort, not longevity, becomes the priority.

Opiates may also cause itching, nausea/vomiting, and constipation.

Diphenhydramine (Benadryl), promethazine (Phenergan), and laxatives/ stool softeners, respectively, are often used to treat these side effects.

- **Morphine.** Probably the best known medicinal narcotic, morphine can be administered in a variety of forms including oral tablets and liquids, intravenous (IV) catheter, intramuscular (IM) injection (a "shot"), and by subcutaneous (under the skin) continuous pump. Hospices tend to use morphine extensively and the subcutaneous continuous pump seems to be used more and more due to certain practical advantages. There are also IV pumps which allow metered, controlled dosing on demand with the push of a button, giving the patient more control.

- **Fentanyl.** An extremely fast acting and rapidly cleared narcotic when given by the IV or IM route. However, fentanyl patches (Duragesic), which slowly release the drug through the skin and usually need replacement every third day, have excellent advantages for end-of-life care. They are very easy and painless to administer by the patient, family, or health care worker. Fentanyl lollipops have also been compounded, allowing the patient to dose his pain control by the amount of time the lollipop stays in his mouth. Children with terminal illnesses are especially well served by this method.

- **Hydromorphone (Dilauded).** A powerful synthetic opiate that is effective for moderate to severe acute pain. Often given by IV or as a rectal suppository in patients in whom IV access is difficult.

- **Darvocet, Percocet, codeine, Lortab, Vicodin, Tylox, Ultram.** These are all oral narcotics of varying strengths that are effective for about four hours. They usually include narcotic and non-narcotic components, although pure forms of the narcotic components can also be prescribed. For the dying patient they may serve as first-line treatment for intermittent mild to moderate pain. They can also be used to treat "breakthrough" pain. For example, if a patient successfully uses Oxycontin (below) for continuous pain relief, she might take an occasional Tylox for pain that "breaks through" occasionally.

- **MS Contin, Oxycontin.** These are long-acting oral opiates. They have received negative publicity beginning in 2001 because of abuse and side effect issues. However, these problems are primarily seen in patients with chronic pain, who are not in the dying process. For the dying patient these medications can provide excellent round-the-clock pain relief with dosing only every twelve hours.

Sedatives

In end-of-life care, medicines from a class called benzodiazepenes (benzo-die-asa-peens) are usually used to prevent or treat restlessness, seizures, anxiety, air hunger (the feeling of not getting enough air into the lungs), and tremors. These medications also increase the effectiveness of actual pain medications. These drugs, in sufficient doses, may also suppress the respiratory drive. Occasionally, they can have an opposite effect and increase agitation, requiring a switch to another agent. As with the opiates, the benzodiazepenes can be addictive, but this is of relatively minor importance in the care of the dying patient.

- **Diazepam (Valium).** Probably the best-known drug in this class, it is long lasting (about twelve hours) and can be given orally, IV, IM, or rectally.

- **Lorazepam (Ativan).** With a shorter onset, it is a good choice for treating seizures that are actively occurring. It lasts only about six to eight hours, so if a patient will be on it long-term, it must be administered more frequently than Valium. The routes of administration are the same as Valium. Seizures are common, unpredictable, and disturbing at the end of life. Often a patient's family or hospice will keep a supply of Ativan suppositories available. If the patient begins seizing, oral, IV, and IM administration may not be possible. The rectal suppository can be placed in almost any situation and usually will control the seizure by the third dose. This treatment can be given at home and may prevent the bystanders from panicking, thereby saving a trip to the emergency department.

AFTERWORD

In closing, we would like to encourage you and your family to initiate a process of dialog, planning, and documentation. There are an infinite number of questions to be answered and many resources available to help you.

This book is a work-in-progress, and our goal is to constantly improve the future editions. It is part of a bigger picture, and we invite you to visit **www.atthecloseofday.com** for updated information and resources. We welcome your feedback and suggestions, which you can provide through the contact information found on the website. Much of the information in this book was included because of suggestions from readers.

If you notice that a new edition of the book comes out after you have bought this one, let us know, and we will e-mail you the new additions.

If this work was helpful to you, please refer people to our website and/or purchase a copy as a gift to help others. If you know of media outlets, medical institutions, or organizations that might have an interest in the book, please let us know so we can expand the vision. We have each spent years working toward improved end-of-life care and are deeply appreciative of your trust and consideration.

—Lance and Bert

Explanation of Terms

Do Not Resuscitate Order (DNR)

Written by a physician, these orders reflect the physician's intent that immediate resuscitation (CPR, ventilation, and other interventions) should not be initiated for a particular patient. This intent may be driven by the physician's belief, and/or the patient/surrogate's belief that such measures are contrary to the patient's best interest due to extremely poor health. DNRs may be included in the hospital or nursing home chart. In most states, a separate DNR form must be signed by a physician and displayed at home for patients whose end-of-life plan includes death at home, in order to prevent EMS personnel who may be called to the scene from beginning resuscitation. Without such documentation, they may be obligated to begin CPR and other measures, even if a living will or surrogate were present. Although it may seem odd to think about a dying patient's surrogate showing EMS a living will and requesting no resuscitation if the patient were to go into cardiopulmonary arrest (a "code"), the reader must remember that without the proper legal document, a good plan may fall apart.

For example, a terminally ill, bed-bound patient may be having intractable pain and needs to be briefly transported to the hospital for better intravenous access so that more pain medicine may be given.

Everyone involved knows the patient may die en route and no one believes CPR would be appropriate. Unless EMS can see the Out-of-Hospital DNR, they may legally have to do just that, even though they feel wrong about it.

Because each state has a different policy regarding out-of-hospital resuscitation by EMS, the details are beyond the scope of this book. Many doctors are not fully aware of this document either and may not have them in the office. However, in order to help you with this additional step we have done research on each state's policy. Initial information is provided at **www.atthecloseofday.com** under "Out-of-Hospital DNR by State." We were amazed by the differences between states and the complexity of some of the policies, but we tried to give you some details and some contact information. We will work to keep the site updated for your convenience.

End-Stage Disease

This term refers to an advanced state of disease. It means the organ systems affected by the disease are failing. For example, if a person has cirrhosis (scarring of the liver), to the point where the liver can no longer function, one would say this person has end-stage liver disease. End-stage dementia would mean this person has a dementia, like Alzheimer's disease. He may have reached a point at which there are no meaningful interactions and is completely incapable of caring for himself. End-stage heart disease means the heart is very weak and is functioning so poorly that it can no longer sustain the body. It can be said that a person with an end-stage disease is in the dying process if no further meaningful interventions can be offered.

Health Care Power of Attorney (HCPOA)

A health care power of attorney allows a person to designate a trusted individual to make health care-related decisions for them in the event they become unable to speak for themselves. The form is similar to, but separate from, a legal power of attorney. For example, a person with a progressive, severe disease might designate an individual as health care power of attorney to deal with her doctors, and then choose a different person as her legal power of attorney to manage estate matters. The two roles can be filled by the same person as well. This document is very powerful in the hands of a trusted individual. Ideally, the person would have a long discussion with her health care power of attorney while she was in a right-minded state, so the health care power of attorney would then have a clear picture of her values and desires in the event of a serious decline of health. Then the health care power of attorney would be able to adapt to a variety of clinical situations, and maintain the patient's values and wishes even in the face of changing situations.

Free copies of state-specific health care power of attorney forms can be downloaded at **www.atthecloseofday.com**.

Hospice

Hospice has slightly different meanings in different areas. A hospice can be a physical institution and place or it can be an organization, or both. Sometimes, a hospice is an actual place where the care given is palliative and comforting rather than interventional and therapeutic. In other words, people go there to die comfortably. Other times, hospice is an organization in the community that sends professionals out to help people die comfortably at home. Again, the main emphasis is that the efforts are toward comfort care, and are not therapeutic. Hospices use medications that alleviate pain and anxiety. They offer spiritual guidance and emotional support, as well as hygiene care and education. A patient's physician can partner with a hospice, but patients can be in hospice without having their own physicians. Most insurance carriers have a hospice benefit, and most hospices have a program for people who are uninsured and unable to pay for their care. Some hospices are associated with religious orders, and some are completely secular. Anyone (health professional, layperson, or patient) may consult hospice. The main acceptance criterion is that a doctor documents an opinion that the patient's life expectancy is reasonably six months or less. More information can be found at the National Hospice and Palliative Care Organization's website, **www.nhpco.org.**

Living Will

A living will is a legal document that varies slightly by state. It is signed and adjusted by the patient to express his desires for care under various circumstances. It usually implies that the patient does not want lifesaving or life-prolonging measures if they are deemed to be in a condition where medical futility has been reached. A living will, when properly presented, would prevent physicians and hospitals from making certain interventions because a patient has already expressed his desire against them. Do Not Resuscitate orders are often associated with living wills. Unfortunately, living wills cannot account for every clinical situation and are sometimes challenged by health care professionals or family members when certain details of a situation were not anticipated in advance.

Free copies of living wills, listed by state, are available at **www.atthe closeofday.com**

Palliative Care

This term is often associated with cancer patients. It basically means that curative attempts will no longer bring advantageous results. The focus then becomes pain control and comfort measures. Hospices often use palliative care as their model.

Notes

Sample Orders

Sample Orders for patient leaving the hospital to die at home.
This is primarily for the health care professional or student.

DISCHARGE TO HOME—
EMS DNR to accompany patient to home bedside.

Diagnosis: End-stage dementia.

Prognosis: Terminal.

Status: Terminal—comfort care only. Do not resuscitate. Do not treat. Do not transport.

No Artificial Hydration or Nutrition.

Diet: Unrestricted, to be offered by family.

Consults: Hospice, ASAP.

Medications: Discontinue all prior medications.

—Morphine Sulphate 4mg intramuscular injection immediately prior to discharge.

—Phenergan 25 mg IM injection immediately prior to discharge.

—Benadryl 12.5 mg IM injection immediately prior to discharge.

—Further pain meds per hospice. [Coordinate with them what you will prescribe for the initial home management, based on their capabilities and your assessment.]

Activity: Bed-bound (or as tolerated if the patient has mobility).

Follow-up: Patient to be followed in home per hospice. Family has appointment in my office tomorrow morning at 9 am.

APPENDIX C

Suggested Reading

These contributions are oriented to professionals who care for the dying.

Ira Byock, *Dying Well: the Prospect for Growth at the End of Life* (Riverbend Books, 1997).
Byock is a physician who has practiced and researched the care of the dying for years and is highly respected as a teacher in this field.

Christine Cassell, ed., *Approaching Death: Improving Care at the End of Life* (The Institute of Medicine, Committee on Care at the End of Life).

Helpful books about the dying process and end-of-life care.

D. J. Enright, ed., *The Oxford Book of Death* (Oxford University Press, 1987).
This is a collection of poems and excerpts from literature on various aspects of death and the views and attitudes reflected in great writing.

Erin T. and Douglas H. Kramp, *Living With the End in Mind* (Three Rivers Press, 1998).
When Erin was diagnosed with a life-threatening illness, they began writing this book, which contains a lot of practical advice and guidance.

Elisabeth Kubler-Ross, *On Death and Dying* (Touchstone, 1997, copyright 1969).
There are several references in the text to this groundbreaking work.

Stephen Levine, *Healing Into Life and Death* (Anchor Books, 1987).
Levine, sometimes working with his wife Ondrea, has published several excellent books with a Buddhist spiritual perspective on the end of life. This one is particularly useful.

JoAnne Lynn et al., *Handbook for Mortals: Guidance for People Facing Serious Illness* (Oxford University Press, 1999).
This book is informative and helps define the state of the art in end-of-life care.

Virginia Morris, *Talking About Death Won't Kill You* (Workman Publishing Company, Inc., 2001).
A layperson talks to the lay reader from outside the medical profession.

George J. Taylor, MD, and Jerome E. Kurent, MD, MPH, *A Clinician's Guide to Palliative Care* (Blackwell Publishing, Inc., 2003).
A clinical perspective for the health care professional or advanced layperson.

Dylan Thomas, "Do Not Go Gentle Into That Good Night," *Poems of Dylan Thomas* (New Directions Publishing Corp., 1952).

Linda Noble Topf, *You Are Not Your Illness* (Fireside, 1995).
While this book is not specifically about terminal illness, it gives wise counsel on keeping one's personal identity separate from the disease or illness one has.

—

In addition to these resources, a number of state or regional hospice organizations have published guides to end-of-life care. Also see our website **www.atthecloseofday.com** for further updates.

ABOUT THE AUTHORS

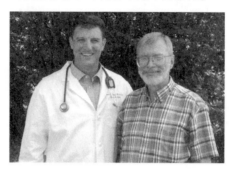

Lance L. Davis, MD, MPH

Lance is a native North Carolinian who currently lives and works in Charleston, South Carolina. He attended the University of North Carolina at Chapel Hill for a Bachelor's of Science in Biology, a Master's degree in Public Health and his Doctor of Medicine. His residency training was in Family Medicine through the Medical University of South Carolina. He is board-certified in Family Medicine, and currently practices Emergency and Family Medicine in the Carolinas. He serves in the U.S. Naval Reserve Medical Corps and is a veteran of Operation Iraqi Freedom. His interest in care of the dying began in medical school and was honed in residency when he began to have responsibility for the care of seriously ill patients. He was mentored by the coauthor, Bert Keller, and is a member of Circular Congregational Church. He has helped guide numerous patients and families through the dying process, and has taught medical students and resident physicians to do the same. Lance enjoys athletics, outdoor activities, the Spanish language and culture, singing, and playing the guitar.

Albert H. Keller, DMin.

Bert was born and grew up in Birmingham, Alabama. He went to Davidson College in North Carolina and Union Theological Seminary in Virginia, spent a year studying theology in France, and earned a Master's degree in Ethics at Yale. His Doctor of Ministry degree is from Princeton Theological Seminary. After teaching for three years in the Congo, Bert came to Charleston, South Carolina to do campus ministry. From that responsibility he moved into the two positions he continues to hold: Associate Professor of Family Medicine (Ethics) at the Medical University of South Carolina and Pastor of Circular Congregational Church (UCC), Charleston. His teaching and research interests are largely in spirituality, the conversation between science and theology, and bioethics. As an outgrowth of teaching doctors and pastoring an active congregation, he was instrumental in organizing the first hospice organization in Charleston (1980) and helping train hospice volunteers. His wife, Lucille, is an actress and theater teacher in a magnet high school. They have three sons.

Keep these pages in mind as you read through the text.
Let them guide you through various stages of planning.

Patient Information

Name of person receiving end-of-life care: _____

Known medical conditions: _____
_____
_____

Current medications:_____
_____
_____

Drug allergies:_____
_____
_____

Health care power of attorney (HCPOA), Name/Telephone:
_____
_____

Family spokesperson (often the same as HCPOA), Name/
Telephone:_____
_____

Primary physician, Name/Telephone:_____

_____

Consulting physicians, Name/Telephone:_____

_____

Hospice, Home Health, and/or Nursing Home, Name/
Telephone: _____

_____

Locations of copies of living will:_____

_____

Locations of copies of health care power of attorney:_____

_____

_____

Locations of EMS/Out-of-Hospital Do Not Resuscitate order
(Some states recommend at the bedside or in the freezer...visit
www.atthecloseofday.com for details): _____

_____

_____

Record of Meetings

This page is provided to help you record the meetings and discussions
that take place with family and/or medical professionals,
and to record hospitalizations. This valuable record will help
to prevent confusion and will keep the plans clear.

DATE   LOCATION   NAMES OF PEOPLE PRESENT   MAJOR POINTS/DECISIONS

General Notes from Reading

Notes

Notes

Notes

Notes

Notes